I was about the biggest skeptic. I had worked at a hospital and heard about the program from a friend who is a licensed physical therapist. I misunderstood the program to be a manipulative procedure and could not understand how an unlicensed person could do this.

I did not understand the stretching concept of this program until I personally had a workout for a hip injury. I had been to my family doctor, took prescription medicine, gone to physical therapy, and was given the option of a cortisone injection into the hip for relief of pain.

A Rossiter trainer encouraged me to try a workout, which I did. I can't begin to tell you how much that first workout helped! This is an effective, hands-on approach to stretching. It gives the employee a feeling of "Wow! This company really cares about me!"

I am now a certified Rossiter trainer and I wholeheartedly recommend it to anyone.

—Linda J. O'Neall, R.N. and occupational health nurse
Creston, Iowa

Before I began using the stretches, my arms would go to sleep from the middle of my neck all the way down to my hands. I had an MRI scan and electrode carpal tunnel testing. Then my arms started falling asleep at night. After I tried and used the Rossiter stretches, I no longer had the deadness in my arms. I can move and work with them now, and they don't go to sleep on me.

—Paula King, inspector
Wauseon, Ohio

I was off work for a repetitive motion injury. It had gotten so bad that I couldn't even grip a doorknob to open it. I couldn't grip my shoelaces to tie them tight. After the fourth Rossiter workout, I could open doors again with my right hand. Now my shoelaces stay tight. Anything's worth a try.

—D.D. Swinford, assembly-line worker
Wauseon, Ohio

I had been injured in a horseback riding accident and had a fractured femur at age twenty-six. One leg was shorter than the other, and it led to degenerative arthritis in the knees. I had so much pain and stiffness I could not do any of my activities. I wasn't able to work as a nurse anymore. If I could walk without pain, I was lucky.

After I had both knees replaced in 1997, I began doing the Rossiter stretches. It made the most remarkable difference in my ability to move. The Rossiter System has made a world of difference. Because of this, I was back at work five weeks after my knee surgery. I tout it every chance I get.

—Sandra R. Wertz, health and safety coordinator
Allentown, Pennsylvania (She danced the conga and Electric Slide at the 1998 Rossiter convention in St. Louis.)

After seventeen years at the same job, I switched jobs. I went from having my hands spread out at work to gripping and holding a power tool. The work involved constant gripping and pressure, and it made my hands hurt so bad. I couldn't hold a telephone or hold on to a steering wheel.

Now I am able to work every day without having surgery, and I don't miss any work. How wonderful! The Rossiter System is very addicting!

—Ralina Cavanaugh, assembly-line worker
Dixon, Kentucky

Overcoming Repetitive Motion Injuries the Rossiter Way

Richard H. Rossiter with Sue MacDonald

Publisher's Note

This publication is designed to provide accurate and authoritative information in regard to the subject matter covered. It is sold with the understanding that the publisher is not engaged in rendering psychological, financial, legal, or other professional services. If expert assistance or counseling is needed, the services of a competent professional should be sought.

Distributed in the U.S.A. by Publishers Group West; in Canada by Raincoast Books; in Great Britain by Airlift Book Company, Ltd.; in South Africa by Real Books, Ltd.; in Australia by Boobook; and in New Zealand by Tandem Press.

Copyright © 1999 by Richard H. Rossiter and Sue MacDonald
      New Harbinger Publications, Inc.
      5674 Shattuck Avenue
      Oakland, CA 94609

Cover design by SHELBY DESIGNS AND ILLUSTRATES

Library of Congress Catalog Card Number: 98-68749
ISBN 1-57224-134-9 Paperback

All Rights Reserved

Printed in the United States of America.

New Harbinger Publications' Website address: www.newharbinger.com

01   00   99

10   9   8   7   6   5   4   3   2   1

First printing

Contents

Part II   The Stretches

Foreword

As an insurance defense attorney, I represent some of the largest insurance companies in Kentucky. I am paid to be skeptical of any health-care provider or system that is outside of the medical community norm.

However, I am always open to any type of therapy or treatment that reduces people's claims of pain, suffering, and loss of power to labor and earn wages. Nonconventional therapies and treatments *must* demonstrate a clear and decisive result before they would be beyond reproach in the courtroom.

With that background, I personally tried the Rossiter System in a half-hearted attempt to relieve the symptoms I suffered from very painful heel spurs, the same condition that plagued basketball great Larry Bird. I admit I was skeptical. After one three-minute session of implementation of Richard Rossiter's System, I was pain-free. I remain pain-free today and am ready to take on Larry Bird one-on-one.

With that kind of result, it's easy to understand how helpful these stretching techniques can be for anyone with aches, pains, or repetitive stress injuries, no matter what their source or cause.

As my grandfather, an Ohio farmer, used to say: "Corn only grows where it's planted." So, too, does the Rossiter System operate: if you use it, you *will* see results. The facts speak for themselves. The Rossiter System gets results—results I would take to the courtroom.

Paul R. Schurman Jr.

Preface

The Evolution of the Rossiter System

By Richard H. Rossiter

I am no stranger to pain. My personal journey through pain, in fact, is what led to the creation of these unique and powerful two-person stretches.

The journey began in Minnesota in high school. During a hockey game, I dislocated my right shoulder. I was an idiot, something I can admit years later. I asked the coach to tape the shoulder together. Bolstered with duct tape and fueled by adrenaline and an attack of being "young and dumb," I went back onto the ice to play hurt. Years later, the injury resurfaced in influential ways.

In the early 1970s, I joined the U.S. Army to learn to fly helicopters. Within months, I was a U.S. Army Warrant Officer and newly trained helicopter pilot assigned to fly search-and-destroy missions out of Quang Tri, South Vietnam.

On April 4, 1971, the OH-58 Kiowa helicopter I piloted was hit by enemy fire in Laos, just across the Vietnamese border. My copilot was killed, and I was forced to land the badly damaged craft.

While waiting to be rescued, the members of my hunt-and-kill team came under "friendly" fire of 500-pound high-altitude bombs that threw up cascading dirt and rocks. The force of falling debris dislocated my left shoulder and broke a spinous process on one of the vertebrae in my back.

Four days later, I was back in the pilot's seat. Later, I was awarded the Bronze Star, the country's third-highest award for valor. (I'm still trying to figure out why I got the medal. For being shot down? Or for being in the right place at the right time to be bombed by my own Air Force?)

During the rest of my nearly yearlong tour of Vietnam, my injured left shoulder began to ache and hurt worse. Flying became more difficult and more painful. The right shoulder, injured during high school hockey, began to ache as well.

After my discharge from the army, I worked as a commercial helicopter pilot. It was during these years of commercial flying that the "minor" hockey injury and the Vietnam injuries began having a major impact. Long days in the pilot's seat were painful for my already achy shoulders. The physical demands and contorted positions required of flying a helicopter added to the misery. (Imagine sitting at a kitchen table with your hands out in front of you, peering under your chair from the side and trying to see the legs on the opposite side of the chair. That's how contorted it was.) Lifting and tilting fifty-five-gallon drums to refuel the craft intensified the aches and pain. Eventually, chronic pain was my constant companion. I couldn't raise my hands above my head.

I began searching for answers.

My search began with the medical profession. Doctors wanted to prescribe painkillers, but the drugs would have limited severely my hours in the air. Since I didn't drink alcohol off-duty because of its effects, prescription drugs were out of the question. The medicines created unpleasant and dangerous side effects, which would be problematic given the difficult and demanding nature of a pilot's job. I couldn't afford to be nauseated, drowsy, dizzy, or confused while flying. My life and the lives of others depended on a clear and sharp mind—mine. It's impossible to land a helicopter on a windy day on a mountain peak in Alaska without being mentally crystal clear. Neither can you gently place from a helicopter into a man's hands five hundred pounds of metal, dangling from a 100-foot line below your helicopter, as he stands atop a 100-foot electrical pole below you.

One surgeon recommended surgery on my shoulder, but he conceded the procedure was risky and held no guarantee of relieving my pain and discomfort. And most people who had undergone surgery told me they were still in pain—it was just a different kind of pain.

I began searching for alternative forms of health care. Eventually, I learned of the Rolf Institute of Structural Integration and other forms of body work, most of which rely on manipulating muscle and/or the body's connective tissue to correct structural and painful problems. Rolfing, specifically, is a form of deep manipulation of the body's connective tissue system. I had heard it was nothing but painful. When I mentioned Rolfing to my medical specialists, they were uninterested at best.

After only three sessions with a certified Rolfer, however, my shoulder pains disappeared. After finishing a full series of sessions, only occasional Rolfing "tune-ups" were needed to keep pain at bay, and I was able to return to flying. I did so with a newfound respect and enthusiasm for Rolfing.

In the 1980s, I applied to the Rolf Institute in Boulder, Colorado, and graduated in near-record time as a certified Rolfer. After establishing a Rolfing practice, first in Austin, Texas, and later in Little Rock, Arkansas, I found I could expand on the concepts of Rolfing to help people identify and stretch through their pain. I also needed to challenge my brain with new ideas. After years of flying a helicopter, coping with everything from treacherous mountain weather to mosquito swarms large enough to carry off my craft, I now found myself in an air-conditioned office with an active, busy practice of fairly predictable problems. Instead of using my brain to combat sheer terror, I studied Rolfing more in-depth and began to examine why Rolfing had been so powerful for relieving the pain in my own shoulders.

One of my clients was a Little Rock neurosurgeon whose back problems I alleviated by using Rolfing techniques. Soon, the doctor began referring a growing number of his patients to me. Some had severe carpal tunnel syndrome. Some were still feeling the effects of surgery that had been performed decades earlier. He sent anyone he thought had any hope of relief. Each person was a special challenge. I could help some, not others, and I began to search for answers. What made the difference between success and failure? What underlying factors were most important in relieving pain and restoring movement or function to the body? What was most effective about Rolfing?

One client was a former factory worker with severe carpal tunnel syndrome. Standard medical treatment for her had included rest, arm and wrist splints, cortisone injections, and two surgeries on her hand. The surgeries left her hand relatively useless, and she continued to experience intense pain from her hand into her neck and head.

Over time, and with the client's willing assistance, I began using, testing, and implementing specific stretching techniques to relieve her pain and restore use to her hand. I integrated my knowledge of connective tissue and other forms of body work and massage. I tried every trick in my body-work bag. I monitored what I did and kept track of what worked.

Gradually, the woman's pain lessened. Hand strength and range of motion returned to her arms. The numbness and tingling she had endured for years eventually disappeared from her hands and arms. Finally, she was free of the symptoms that had caused her years of suffering.

Elated by her recovery, I began applying these newfound and newly evolved stretching techniques to other clients referred by the same neurosurgeon. I discovered that many people responded almost immediately to these techniques. Instead of months of treatment and repeated sessions, many people achieved lasting pain relief after only a few stretching workouts. For most, only occasional "tune-up" sessions were needed to remain virtually free of symptoms and pain.

In time, I set out to create a simplified but highly teachable system of stretches to help the millions of people who are victims of carpal tunnel syndrome, repetitive motion injuries, and other common types of body aches and pains. The Rossiter System techniques are simple, effective, and highly efficient.

For ten years, the Rossiter System has been adopted in factories, industries, and businesses to help employees work more productively and pain-free and to hold down rising medical bills and worker's compensation claims from on-the-job injuries, pain, and disability. Many of the companies using the Rossiter System experience dramatic reductions in medical and worker's compensation costs—and rising rates of productivity and satisfaction among workers. Now these stretches are being made available to the general public.

I developed these stretches to get rid of my own pain and the pain of others. I am passionate about them, and I hope you will be, too. It is immensely satisfying to see people who are crippled by pain walk away from these stretches with a sense of hope, power, and renewed mobility.

More than anything, I hope you find the joy and freedom I've found in becoming pain-free. Your problems may not disappear entirely, but they'll be easier to handle because you'll be out of pain. And if and when they do recur (and they will, if you live on Planet Earth), you will be able to give a repeat performance and stop the pain once again.

My Part in the Rossiter System

By Sue MacDonald

In more than twenty years as a newspaper journalist, I've written about thousands of topics and interviewed as many people. None of them inspired me to write a book until I met Richard H. Rossiter.

Of course, it helped tremendously that in the course of a one-hour interview, he fixed a sore shoulder that had plagued me for months. My shoulder pain is an occupational hazard—the result of perching a telephone receiver in the crook of my neck for more than twenty years while typing at a computer. (I now use a telephone headset and the Rossiter stretches religiously.)

But I really found out how effective these stretches were when Richard accepted an invitation to the annual Thanksgiving get-together at my parents' house. By the end of the evening, he had "fixed" the sore hips, aching backs, tender shoulders, shin pain, elbow tendinitis, and various other bodily ailments of a steady stream of cousins, sisters, in-laws, and friends. They were a cross section of people in pain—a computer programmer, a nurse, an aerobics student, a teacher, a truck driver, a retired office secretary, a farmer.

"When can we buy your book?" they all asked, and that's when I knew it was time for the book that was always hidden inside this writer to come out and meet the world.

By the nature of my profession, I am a skeptic. I must see to believe. These stretches have made me a believer. I do them with my children (for their softball, basketball, viola-playing, and computer aches) and they do them with me (daily stress, computer aches, shoulder/neck pain).

One of the joys of my job is hearing feedback from readers who say, "Thanks, you helped me" or "I never knew that before" or "You made me think about something differently." These stretches will do the same for you—make you think and act differently to get rid of your pain.

When you run across the pronoun "I" in this book, it's Richard talking. This is his work, and these are his ideas. I'm just flattered to be the conduit through which these ground-breaking stretches reach the general public.

Sometimes, ideas and people rattle around in this world waiting for the right time to meet, mesh, and otherwise find each other. This is one of those times. And after more than twenty years as a professional writer, I'm proud to claim this as a first book.

Acknowledgments

First, I want to thank Sandi Shade for her tireless effort to bring the first full Rossiter program into an industrial setting. I want to thank her, too, for the years of love and friendship she brought to my life.

I'd like to thank Donna Stone, or rather Donna Brown, newly married. We now like to think of her as Donna Brownstone. Donna has kept me going for almost ten years by pushing and goading me. She's my best friend and confidant.

Without Sue MacDonald, there wouldn't be a book. I'm thrilled to have met her. She put up with my head turning red after reading first drafts of what she thought I'd said. Patience is her middle name, or it ought to be.

I want to thank Kenn Spencer for inspiration on a daily basis. I want to thank Mary Niepling and Judy Stacy for their constant rereading of the manuscript, making sure it was readable for anyone. I want to thank everyone in my office, including Carolyn Ascher for her creative input into all our materials. Thanks to Bill Tilson for his doggedness at staying the course.

Special thanks to wordsmith and friend Kathy Doane, and to graphic design wizard Ron Huff, for making the book proposal look so good that a publisher nibbled and bit. And more thanks to artists Randy Mazzola and Jim Borgman, both of whom continue to amaze with their talents.

To all who reviewed the manuscript and offered advice, thanks for your professional input. To the doctors who returned phone calls and answered questions about anatomy, drugs, surgery, and other topics, thanks for your kindness and insight: Dr. Thomas G. Saul, neurosurgeon, Mayfield Clinic & Spine Institute, Cincinnati, Ohio; Dr. Timothy E. Kremchek, orthopaedic surgeon and sports medicine specialist, Cincinnati, Ohio; Dr. Pamela Schurman, osteopathic surgeon, Pace, Fla.; Cincinnati Drug & Poison Information Center Staff; Dr. David Dahlman, chiropractor and nutritionist, Cincinnati, Ohio.

Thanks to Sara and Tim Bedinghaus for sharing the computer. The world should have more teenagers like you.

And to all who offered encouragement, support and go-get-'ems over the years, thanks for your friendship and spirit.

I'd also like to thank Evan, because she brings joy to my life, even far away.

In memory of Chief Warrant Officer Peck, a lost friend from Vietnam whose life sacrifice made this book possible.

Thanks again, Sue. I love you.

Richard H. Rossiter

Introduction

Step Out
of Pain

If you picked up this book because you're in pain, good for you. For the first time in weeks, months, or even years, you will learn how to chase pain out of your body for good. Without pills, shots, awkward splints or surgery, you will gain power over your pain using nothing more than natural healing powers within your own body and its connective tissue. All you need is an understanding of how the pain got where it is, a partner to help you stretch, and the willingness to find the pain in your body and get rid of it.

It's unfortunate that you're in pain; but the pain is there for a reason. Owning your pain is the first step to getting rid of it. If you own it, you can disown it, and the Rossiter System will show you how to do so naturally. This book is about stepping away from pain pills, tissue-destroying shots, or disabling surgeries that don't really make your pain go away. These stretches will put you in step with thousands of other people who use them to resume activities and jobs and remain pain-free.

The Rossiter stretches are based on the seventy-year-old concepts of a form of body work called Rolfing as well as on other massage techniques. The Rossiter System stretches evolved over ten years of working with people in severe pain, and now they're being used nationwide by thousands of people with great success. These stretches are based on solid information. They are not 100 percent effective for everyone, but they are practical, simple, and easy to learn.

Will you be officially pain-free for life? Of course not. But when you get in a bind, you'll have a quick solution and you'll have control. You won't have to wait out the pain. You won't have to wait for a doctor's appointment. You'll be able to get out of pain with the help of only a friend.

Perhaps you're suffering from carpal tunnel syndrome, a backache, a sore shoulder, a stiff neck, achy hands, or arm pain. There are thousands of ways for your body to get sore from working, playing, and everyday living. Maybe you have constant headaches. Maybe you ache or are numb from typing, cutting, chopping, lifting, sitting in one position, driving, doing aerobics, pushing, pulling, using power tools, repeating the same task hundreds of times a day, or performing weekend-warrior athlete heroics. Take your pick. If you are in pain, you're certainly not alone.

In 1995, the U.S. Bureau of Labor Statistics found that 62 percent of all workplace injuries in the mid-1990s were caused by *repetitive stress*—repeating the same task or motion. *Carpal tunnel syndrome*, a disabling injury of the wrist and hand, was the most common and was responsible for the most work-related absenteeism.

Repetitive-stress disorders, also called repetitive motion injuries (RMI) or cumulative trauma disorders (CTD), sap an estimated $100 billion from the U.S. economy through sick days, lowered productivity, and employee retraining. And that study examined only work-related injuries. Many people experience pain, injury, and limited mobility from recreational sports, hobbies and the simple activities of daily life.

How Does the Rossiter System Work?

If you've been to a doctor, physical therapist, chiropractor, or specialist for your pain, you've probably been told the muscles are pulled or strained. Maybe you've been told the ligaments in your wrist are squeezing the nerves and your only hope is to cut them surgically to free the nerves. Maybe you've been told that swelling and inflammation in your tissues need to be treated with anti-inflammatory medicines, cortisone shots, painkillers, and muscle relaxants.

The real truth is this: Drugs dull pain and hide it from you; they do not take it away. Splints and braces trap pain and eventually send it somewhere else to make its presence felt. Cortisone, over time, will weaken and destroy tissue, which is why doctors limit its use. Surgery cuts vital, living tissue that these stretches can repair.

The Rossiter System stretches and techniques laid out in this book will give you control of your pain, teach you how to work it out of your body, and help you keep it out for good. How? They stretch out the connective tissue that's causing you to hurt right now.

"What is connective tissue?" you might be wondering. Not something you recall from biology class, is it? Probably not. *Connective tissue* is the network of protective sheaths, tendons, ligaments, fascia, and cartilage that holds your body together, from the tip of your toes to the top of your head, and gives it shape.

What's happening in your body right now is a physical insult to the connective tissue that holds your body together. Your body is sending you a powerful message: "This is not right. This body hurts. Fix me."

Normally, connective tissue allows your body to move freely and fluidly. It holds you together. It is the thin-but-strong tissue that wraps around individual cells and entire muscles, the stretchy bands that tie muscles, bones, and joints together. But because of injury or repeating the same motion over and over, your connective tissue has thickened. It's become shorter than it should be. It's holding you together too tightly. It's as if your body, once a long, loose rope, has become twisted, knotted, and kinked, the way a phone cord kinks when it's twisted too much. When working or playing, connective tissue should be ready to use, like the rope in figure 1. Not taut, but almost. It has a little tension. Just like your connective tissue, the rope in figure 2 starts to knot up when stressed. The place of a kink is where you'll feel pain (say, in a wrist or elbow), but the entire area will have tension. The kink starts at the weakest or most overworked area, and it spreads from there, taking pain with it.

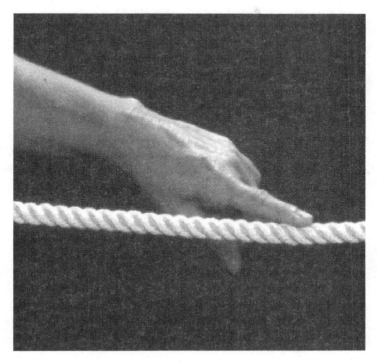

Figure 1   Normal Connective Tissue

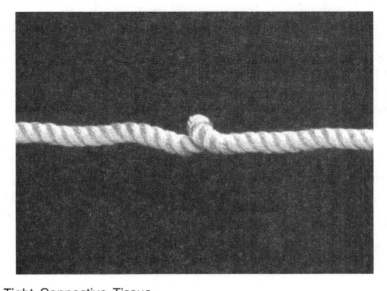

Figure 2   Tight Connective Tissue

Connective tissue under those circumstances can't take in nutrients or oxygen properly, so it's starving, shortening, and hurting. When the connective tissue wrapping of your muscles and nerves is crimped, your muscles and nerves are not getting the food and fuel they need to carry on normal activity. You'll read more about connective tissue in chapter 2.

The Rossiter System offers a fix that lasts. It doesn't cover or hide the pain the way over-the-counter and prescription painkillers do. It doesn't force the pain to stay in a flat position or inside a splint. It doesn't cut out the pain with a surgeon's scalpel.

The Rossiter System stretches return connective tissue to its normal state—mobile, loose, and supple—because they target connective tissue specifically and stretch it out. Remember, connective tissue is squeezing and limiting the space between your muscles and your bones. That's why you hurt and are in pain.

In a matter of minutes after a Rossiter workout, the numbness and tingling of carpal tunnel syndrome in your wrists (or pain and stiffness in your shoulders, neck, arms, or back) will respond to the exercises and stretches laid out for you in this book. That's right—in a matter of minutes, your pain will start to ease, and it will stay away for days or weeks. More importantly, you will have the tools to keep it out of your body for the rest of your life. The Rossiter System has been successful in numerous American factories because results are achieved in a matter of minutes, not days or weeks. Workers who hurt and undergo these stretches often feel better in twenty to thirty minutes and can go right back to work. You can have that same success, too.

The Rossiter System in Action

You may be skeptical. Many people are when they first learn of these two-person stretches and this approach. It's probably unlike anything you've ever seen or tried. The techniques may even look a little strange.

But thousands of American factory and office workers have been using these stretching workouts for ten years to alleviate most upper-body structural pain. They do it on the job—in workout rooms inside factories or in conference rooms set up with protective floor mats. Some workers often are skeptical at first. But all it takes is a demonstration. Try it on yourself. Practice with a friend, spouse, or partner (you'll get a really easy try-me opportunity in chapter 1). You'll be amazed.

Here are some stories of people who tried the Rossiter System and benefited from its effects:

Gary Jackson, factory worker

"Physical" doesn't come close to describing Gary Jackson's job. He works as a "turner" for a garment company that makes men's coats. Several thousand times a day, he slips his arms into the loose lining of a coat, pulls it inside out, slips the lining into the outer shell and sleeves of the coat, then flips, or turns over, both layers of material—sometimes heavy denim or thermal linings—so the coat parts can be sewn together.

"It's a very physical job. It takes a lot of upper-body work, and it's a very, very tiresome job," says Jackson, thirty-seven, who has been a turner for five years. After only a few months on the job, he began to feel the harsh effects of doing the same labor-intensive job, hour after hour, day after day. "My shoulders would hurt, and then I'd hurt underneath my collarbone," he says. "It gave me some awesome pain just to lift my arm up."

A doctor told him the arm was worn out. A physical therapist prescribed exercises that didn't really help. When his employer instituted the Rossiter System in 1994, Gary began attending twice-weekly stretching sessions.

"I really hurt before I began the Rossiter program," he says. "But after a few weeks of doing the stretches, I noticed a tremendous difference. Now I can go in to the Rossiter room and stretch out—and I don't hurt. I basically go now for maintenance, because the everyday pain is gone. It's a great program. I believe in it. . . . If I had to stand there and hurt like I once did, there's no way I could continue doing my job."

Beverly Wild, customer service representative

For most of her life, Beverly Wild has worked at computers. Now fifty-six and a customer service representative for a Cincinnati welding supply wholesaler, she began experiencing thumb pain and numbness in her arm at night in late 1997. "I've also had off-and-on headaches since high school," Beverly says. Most of her workday is spent on the telephone and entering data into a computer.

She began doing the Rossiter stretches with her husband in late 1997. In three weeks, feeling had returned to her arms, and the thumb pain dissipated. Better yet, she quit taking Advil daily. "My extreme headaches also went away—and they involved pain that I felt from my jaw all the way into my head at times," she says. "Whatever these stretches did, they took the pain away."

Mary Ophelia Alatorre, printer

Until she began using Rossiter System stretches, Mary Ophelia Alatorre went home every night with swollen knuckles after only a month on the job at a magazine bindery and printing plant in Pennsylvania. She works as a pocket filler, pushing and positioning pages of magazine sections into grids, or "pockets," so they can be compiled with other gridded sections before being bound together as a single magazine.

Because of the hand pain, she was assigned to lighter duty at work, attended physical therapy sessions for several months, and made a weekly visit to the company doctor. But the pain and swelling in her hands persisted, even after three or four days of rest.

In April, 1997, her employer, installed the Rossiter System. "I was one of those nonbelieving people," Mary says. "I went into it thinking, 'Well, it can't hurt, but it's probably not going to help.'

"Now, I'm a believer. After the Rossiter workouts, the swelling will go down right away. And if I keep up with the stretches several times a month, it keeps the swelling down.

"I've told people they'll probably be skeptical about it. Initially it might cause some soreness because you don't know you have those muscles that are sore. But it's a good kind of sensation. It just makes you want to go right back to work."

How to Use This Book

This book will help you in two ways. Part 1 explains the structural reasons and causes for chronic pain, helps you understand why your body hurts, and provides you with information about how and why these stretches relieve pain. Part 2 is the meat and potatoes of the Rossiter System. It provides step-by-step instructions for learning the basic stretches to relieve upper-body pain and low back pain. By learning these stretches, you'll be able to get rid of pain, numbness, and tingling in your thumbs, fingers, hands, wrist, arm, elbow, shoulders, neck, head, face, and lower back.

It's possible for you to jump from this chapter directly to the stretches. If that's what you want to do—jump! But if you want background information, keep reading until you get to the stretches. (My guess is you'll eventually read the entire book, but it's up to you how to start.)

However, I must ask you to read the chapters about back pain and how it develops before doing the back stretches. It's for your own safety that you read those first.

Please read about, practice, and learn these stretches with an open mind. They are unconventional. They're going to hurt at times, but the hurt will be good because it will be rousting the pain away from your connective tissue and into thin air.

You will never feel the same again. You will feel better. You will feel freer. You will feel lighter. You will be happier because your mind will no longer be plagued and harangued by endless, grating, ever-present nagging pain.

See for yourself, and then you'll be hooked. Good luck! I know you can do this.

Part I

About the Rossiter System

Chapter 1

Ouch! Taking Control of Pain Before It Takes Control of You

Pain. The mere whisper of the word causes you to wince, doesn't it? There's no need to state the obvious, but pain hurts. If you're a parent who has stepped on a high-heeled Barbie shoe or tiny Lego in the middle of the night, you know instant pain. If you're a factory worker who lifts the same heavy boxes or uses the same power tool thousands of times a day, you know chronic pain. If you're sore from aerobics or talking on the phone with a receiver crooked in your shoulder, you know nagging, dull, always-there pain. Pain is something everyone feels, but not everyone understands it.

Pain exists for a reason. Pain is a message. Pain is information. It's your body's intercom system setting off red blinking lights and buzzers and yelling, "This does not feel good! Something is wrong! Stop doing that! Fix this!" It is your body's way of telling you things are out of whack, overused, injured, or stressed out.

Moreover, if pain is ignored, it eventually grows, buzzes, and yells louder.

Pain can work its way into your body subtly or it can have an obvious cause, such as twisting at the waist while lifting something heavy. Regardless of how pain got into your body, the time has come for you to work pain out of your body using the Rossiter System.

Getting Rid of Your Pain: The Deer-Hunting Analogy

Maybe it's because I'm from Minnesota, but I frequently use a deer-hunting analogy to make my point (no offense to Bambi). Let's say you're a hunter who is going out to bag some deer. (Without being sexist or politically incorrect, I know that some readers may not identify with the deer-hunting concept, so if you're one of those readers, when you see the words "hunt deer," insert the phrase "shop for shoes." It's the same principle.)

First, would you go downtown to set up your deer stand? Of course not. It's ridiculous to hunt where there are no deer. Okay, so you move the deer stand into the woods, and then you calmly take out a blindfold and cover your eyes. Right? Certainly not. You need to be able to see what you're hunting.

Suppose you climb into the deer stand and then tie one of your hands to the tree. It's not tied tightly, just enough to restrict your movement. Will it do you any good to be in an advantageously placed deer stand with one hand unable to move? No, of course it won't.

Did I mention your gun? It's a bazooka, and it's very effective at blowing things to smithereens. Not necessarily good for hitting a deer precisely, but it gets the job done, even if it's not quite the job you had in mind.

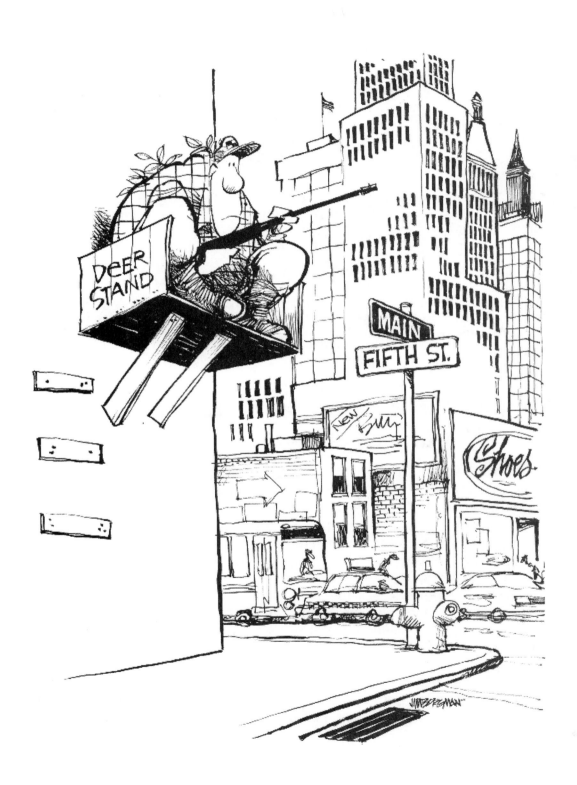

Lastly, when you see the deer, should you turn around immediately and make sure the animal is behind you? Isn't it better to shoot when you can't see it? Of course not.

Here's my point about deer hunting and pain: If you don't go after your pain in the right area, with the right tools, in the right way, you will not get the results you need or want. If you understand all these points, you'll understand the who, how, where, and why of getting rid of your pain.

Who

Just as it's the hunter's responsibility to track the deer, it's your responsibility to track and own your pain. No one else can fix it for you. Blaming it on someone else, or expecting someone else to fix it, simply won't work because it's your body and your pain. Only you live in your body.

How

When hunting for pain, painkillers, anti-inflammatory medicines, muscle relaxants, and shots are like big fat mittens that don't allow you to feel anything. They dull your senses to the pain. Your body is trying to tell you something, and those drugs are saying, "Shut up. See? Feel? It's not here." Just as a hunter cannot wear a blindfold into the woods or meadow, you need to remove the mittens to sense, identify, and fix the pain.

Likewise, tying your hand to a tree restricts your movement. It makes you an ineffective hunter. When you put your hand or wrist in a splint or brace, you diminish your ability to move.

As for weaponry, a bazooka certainly isn't the approach you want. Shoot a bazooka at a deer, and you'll have deer burger. If you overdo your approach to relieving pain—and surgery is perhaps the ultimate example of overdoing the idea of pain control—you can't reap the rewards of the hunt because you're overdoing it.

Just because your pain is located in a certain or specific spot (your wrist, for example), that doesn't make your wrist the enemy. The wrist is only the weakest link or the victim, and beating up on victims is useless. It doesn't solve the problem, and it just lets the bad guy (your pain) free to come back and victimize again. (And if pain returns to your wrist after surgery, then what?)

Where

Setting up a deer stand at Fifth and Main, or even in the wrong area of the woods, is stupid at worst and careless at best. (Likewise, hunting for shoes in the woods is silly. Everyone knows you go to the mall). When dealing with pain, you have to find its source, not focus on the result. That's why I hammer home the importance of hunting for pain inside your body. You're the hunter, and you're after the source of your pain.

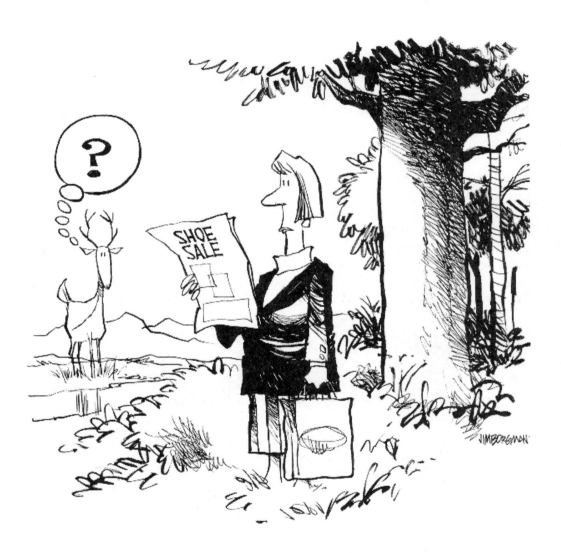

Why

Getting rid of pain is your main objective. It's what you want the most—to keep the nagging, aching, and sheer pain out of your body. You want to get rid of your pain with no bad consequences. That means you can't aim at your pain with bazookas, shots, or surgery, because they all inherently have negative consequences.

You need an appropriate weapon against pain, one that makes you a successful hunter without making deer burger of your own body. Your goal should be to stretch your body's connective tissue system back to its normal state, because doing so gets rid of your pain.

Start Your Own Pain Hunt Right Now

Are you ready to begin relieving your pain?

Try this quick demonstration: Find a spot on your arm and grab it between the thumb and forefinger of your opposite hand. Hold it tightly. (See figure 1.1.) Make it hurt a bit so you know you're holding tightly enough. But don't squeeze so hard that you can't keep the pressure even. Notice what happens to the pain the longer you maintain your hold. First, the tissue under your fingers softens. Second, the pain dulls under your fingers. That's pain moving out of the area. Remember how your mom would rub a sore area to make the pain go away? Or how you do it to yourself when something hurts? The Rossiter System is the same concept, but it's applied strategically.

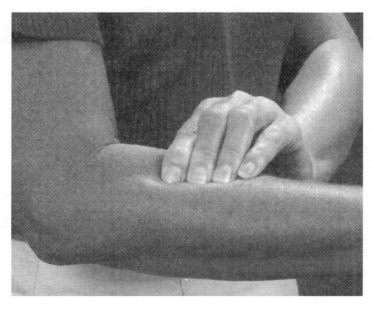

Figure 1.1   Squeeze and Hold

That's the essence of these stretches—by applying weight as you stretch, you soften connective tissue so it can stretch out, and by stretching connective tissue, you make pain go away. It's that simple. The Rossiter stretches are conscious fixes for pain. The amount of relief you get depends on how willing you are to go after the pain in your body and chase it out.

Pain is a nasty master. It changes who you are, day to day. Each day you stay in pain, you affect people around you. Perhaps you've seen it in your own family—a mother who eats pills all day or a father who lies on the couch constantly with a bad back (and an equally nasty temperament!). Many people take their pain out on others. It's easier than taking charge of it.

Go Out the "In" Door

The Rossiter stretches allow you—empower you—to be in charge of your pain. The pain is yours, and so is the power to rid it from your body. Granted, facing pain isn't easy, but avoiding pain always makes it worse. There is only one way out of pain, and that is the way you came in. You are the only specialist, the only expert, about your own pain. Nobody's pain is like your pain. Only you can find your way out.

To describe this concept, I often use the image of five people in the Room of Pain. Each person has a different place in this room. They all look around and see that there's one door and a few chairs around, each chair a different distance from the door. Everyone knows they came in through the door. Everyone understands and accepts that the door is the only way out.

However, when people are in pain, they often want relief *right now*. They don't want to walk all the way across the room to the door, because it hurts to walk that far. Some take pills or pursue altered states of mind that make them feel they're not in the room. Some will sit on the chairs, not moving anything, in hopes of not upsetting the pain (which is similar to wearing a splint or staying in bed). Some will resort to drilling and blasting—blowing out the roof, wall, or floor—to get out. Some will wait for someone else to come and rescue them.

Or they could all go out the way they came in—through the door. What a novel idea!

These stretches provide the help you need to get out of pain so that you don't hurt yourself in the process. These stretches help you get to the door and get out of the Room of Pain.

All you need is some assistance, nothing more. It's that simple. In East Asian cultures, the highest form of healing is by one who touches another. By teaming with a partner to get rid of your pain, you're combining two powerful forces—self-empowerment and human touch.

You are the hero of this stretching program. You must be willing to grunt and groan and pull the pain out of your body. If it comes back, go in and get it again. If it changes places, size, or feeling, get it again. Smack that sucker! Get mad! Go after your pain with all the guts and mustard you have.

After a workout, you may feel a little sore. You might hurt. You may wince or cringe a lot. You may break into a sweat or cry. It's like any workout at any gym or aerobics class. You'll be glad when you're done.

That's good. That's okay. Especially with structural pain, feeling the hurt means you've found your pain and are helping it find its way out of your body.

Compensating for Pain

Finding pain inside the body can sometimes be tricky, because people in pain often compensate. If doing certain movements hurt, they'll change the movements slightly. They'll slouch or shift their weight. They'll rely more heavily on body parts that don't hurt in order to compensate for the parts that do. They'll back off a heavy workload or slack off on effort.

It's a bugaboo to every person who experiences chronic pain. Compensating for pain can send it somewhere else in the body without your even realizing what's happened. Compensation has serious effects because people often compensate instinctively or unconsciously, unaware of how or why they've tried to give pain the old runaround. But believe me, if you give pain the runaround, it will sneak back and run all over you.

I've noticed some common scenarios over the years while talking to people about traumatic or repetitive motion injuries.

Scenario One: "Well, it used to hurt here," someone will say, pointing to a spot on the hand or wrist, "and then it began to hurt over here [pointing to an elbow], and now this is the spot that really bothers me" [indicating a shoulder].

Scenario Two: "Well, now that you've worked on my shoulder for the last hour, I just remembered that what started all this pain wasn't in my shoulder at all. It was actually some discomfort in my neck and upper arm that first bothered me a few years ago, but the shoulder pain is what brought me to your office for help."

The same kinds of stories are told by all sorts of people. Here's what usually happens. Let's say an assembly-line worker notices a pain while she's working. As the pain becomes more intense, she changes the way she executes a specific task. Usually, it's not a big change, just a slight adjustment in how she performs the work. If the pain stops, she continues doing the task the new way. The original source of the pain could have been an aerobics or job-related injury, but it doesn't matter because now it's a second-generation pain that's been covered up by a first-generation compensation. Welcome to the world of compensations!

Usually, the compensation is unconscious, and the person doesn't know she's doing a particular task differently. She's just doing the job the best she can. Then the pain strikes again.

"How'd you get that pain?" I'll ask.

"I don't know. I've been doing this job for twenty years," is a common reply.

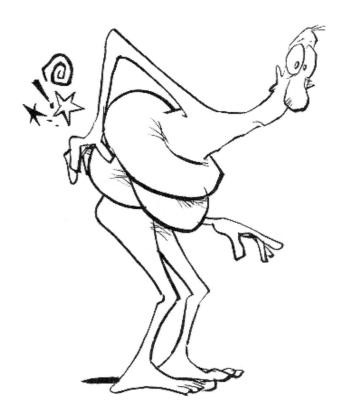

In actuality, the job hasn't stayed the same for twenty years. It changed when the worker first experienced pain. At that moment, she altered some small aspect of the work that probably wouldn't be noticeable to anyone else. Yet now she's in pain, after all these years. Perhaps it's a pain in the shoulder that's evident now, but over the intervening years, she's forgotten about the original pain because the latest compensation has moved the pain elsewhere. Third- and fourth-generation compensations for pain can produce achiness all over. Over time, the effects of the compensations accumulate (which is why chronic pain is often called cumulative trauma disorder). Sound familiar?

As you begin to do these stretches, it's likely you'll discover and uncover a long list of complaints, a series of body parts or sites that hurt, ache, and throb. What you're doing is unwinding all those pent-up traumatic incidents or compensations, like peeling layers off an onion. Each layer stings and makes your eyes water, but at different intensities.

Remember, you have years and years of new and old pains, compensations, and information embedded in your body. With these stretches, you'll systematically unravel, uncover, and deal with all those injuries and all that pain.

Uncovering and healing pain is a normal part of these stretches. With a stretching partner, you systematically will work out the body kinks that are both obvious and hidden. Eventually the compensations unwind and the body will return to a normal, healthy state.

Believe this: these stretches may hurt, but they produce a good hurt. Why? It's a hurt that goes away. It's a temporary hurt or residual pain from the stretching you've just done. This isn't sharp, stinging pain. Rather, you'll feel the pain relief of tissue that's been stretched, loosened, and worked out. Because a certain area of your body has been cramped and tight for so long, moving it freely now will feel a little new and untried. But it will feel better.

You will feel so good at the end of the first stretching session that you will scarcely believe it. Your arms will feel light and floaty. They will move freely, not disjointedly or slowly. All that hidden pain will be exorcised. Even the shape of your body will change: your shoulders will elongate a few millimeters, and they may rest a bit lower, more relaxed, instead of being pulled upward. Take a good look at your body now, and compare it to your body after a stretching workout. You'll see the difference. As you become better at stretching the effects are even more pronounced.

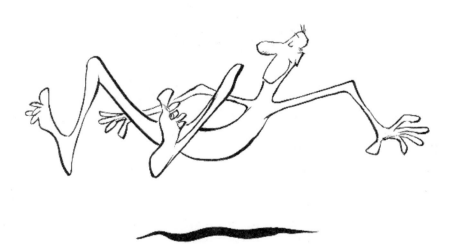

The difference is most noticeable if you stop during a workout after stretching just one side of your body. Look in a mirror and compare the stretched side with the unstretched side. Take a good look at the slope of your shoulders, and notice how relaxed the stretched side is.

By comparing and consciously stretching, you'll see pain leave your body. Once you can see and produce results, you'll know how to get rid of pain wherever and whenever it returns.

When I worked as a Rolfer, clients would sometimes walk around the room to rest between stretches. I would notice a difference in how their bodies looked and moved and would frequently tell them so. Most thought I was a little crazy until I'd stand them in front of a mirror and let them see the change too. They'd become excited. They'd want to continue with the stretching techniques. It's uplifting to see positive results from hard-fought changes in life. It's especially exciting when the results are immediate and tangible. There's no waiting for results with the Rossiter techniques. These stretching workouts will give you a sense of accomplishment.

If you're in pain, this is your wake-up call, and you can answer it or pretend not to hear it. My sincere hope is that you answer resoundingly. It will not be easy, but few things worthwhile ever are.

Chapter 2

Connective Tissue: The Key to the Rossiter System

Living in northern Minnesota, I know a lot about hunting. So, the first time friends told me about connective tissue, they described skinning a deer. They talked about the shiny, silky stuff under the skin and between the muscles—threadlike sheets they have to remove to get to the meat. This iridescent sheathlike tissue lined the cavity of the deer. It weaves in and out of all the muscles, tendons and ligaments. Some of it is almost clear. Other parts are thick and opalescent. The thickest connective tissue is white and bright. All of it was slick and beautiful. It may sound a little gross, but this is the best way to describe what connective tissue looks like.

What Is Connective Tissue?

Connective tissue is really quite simple to understand. It does exactly what it sounds like it does: it connects every part in the body to all the other parts. It connects bones to bones, muscles to bones, muscles to muscles. You've probably heard it referred to by other names—cartilage, ligaments, and tendons.

Connective tissue has subparts with names like epimesium, perimesium, and endomesium. They are specific components of cartilage, ligaments, and tendons. That's as technical as this book gets. In fact, the technical term I'll use from now on when referring to connective tissue's parts or subparts is *stuff*.

Having a hard time visualizing connective tissue? Think of it as a long, thin, strong rope that stretches from the tip of your head to the bottom of your toes. All along its length, it holds together muscles, bones, joints, organs, and anatomical stuff. Each and every cell has a layer of connective tissue around it (see figure 2.1). Small groups of cells are swathed in it, and so are larger groups. Tiny muscle strands are wrapped in it, and so are entire groups of muscles.

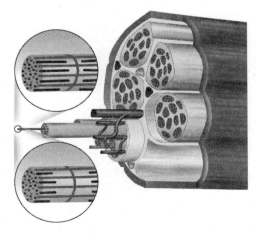

Figure 2.1   Connective Tissue Surrounds Muscles as They Contract and Relax

Inside the body, in fact, connective tissue looks like a multi-layered gossamer sheet (see figure 2.2), so thin in some areas it is translucent and so thick in others it is opaque. When you trim a raw steak or eat a cooked steak and find that whitish sheet of stretchy thin tissue between natural sections of meat, that's connective tissue. If you pull apart the meat sections, you'll notice even thinner pieces of stuff stuck to the meat. It's all various forms of connective tissue. Another name for this tissue is *fascia* (pronounced FASH-ya).

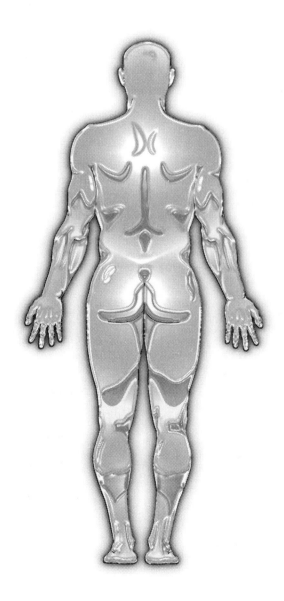

Figure 2.2 The Gossamer Body

Here's another way to think about it: Imagine that I came to your home and started Saran-Wrapping all your dishes, one at a time, with one long sheet of wrap. Each plate and cup would be encircled and returned to its original spot. Then with the same piece of wrap, I would wrap your table, your couch, your bed, your entire house, inside and out. Mind you, nothing would be wrapped tightly. Everything simply would be wrapped and enclosed inside one, long piece of flexible film.

Think the Saran-Wrapping is finished? Not yet. Next I would walk to the house next door and start wrapping the neighbor's dishes, couch, table, entire house—and then the entire street, until the whole neighborhood was wrapped. Power lines, sewage pipes, telephone wires, cars and trucks, parks, water lines, highways, streets. Everything would be wrapped. Remember, this is all done with the same piece of plastic wrap flowing in the same general direction. Got the picture?

Next, both ends would be stretched to the nearest road overpass—that would be the same as the bones in your body—and bolted there. Then the wrapping process would move to the next neighborhood and be repeated.

Now, ask yourself this: What if the entire community couldn't exist without this special wrap? What if everything fell apart and out of place without it? What if everything would leak and tumble without this protective, stretchy enclosure? What if connective tissue was just as important to your body as the air you breathe?

Simple Try-Me Exercises

The introduction promised a simple activity to prove how the body's connective tissue ties your anatomy together, from the tip of your toes to the top of your head. Here it is: Find a partner and a chair. Have your partner sit in the chair, with both arms hanging loosely at his or her sides. Ask your partner to sit up straight, feet flat on the floor. Both of you take deep breaths and relax. Now, gently place your thumb and the fingerprint part of your forefinger on the hard, bony surface just below the bridge of your partner's nose. Use a light, gentle touch. Pretend you're holding a grape. Don't squish it.

Now, ask your partner to start a long, slow wiggle with one hand (it doesn't matter which one), like a gentle wave. Have your partner stretch out the fingers and vary the speed of the hand and finger movements. It should be done slowly. The partner's arm and shoulder should not move—just the fingers and hand should be in motion.

As you hold the bridge of the person's nose, what do you feel? Anything? Something? Most likely, you'll feel a subtle yet definite movement under your fingertips. How subtle? It's almost like tiny threads moving back and forth. It may feel as if something is sliding or rolling. Now change places with your partner and do the same exercise.

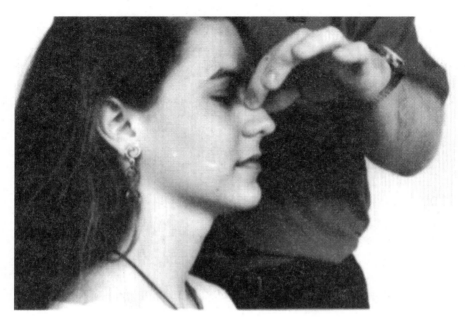

Figure 2.3   Nose Grip

Don't talk during the process. Feel. If you talk, you won't feel, because the vibrations of your speech will muffle the threadlike sensation under your fingertips.

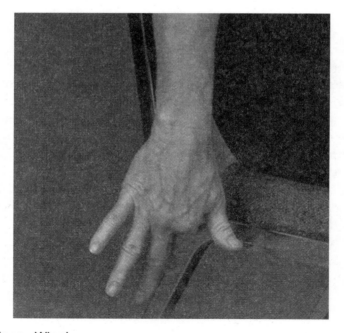

Figure 2.4   Finger Wiggle

Keep practicing on each other. Try wiggling the fingers with varied speeds. Move the fingers slowly then faster, and be aware of the different sensations at the bridge of the nose with each speed.

Don't worry if you don't feel anything right away. With practice, you will. It takes only a few minutes to get the hang of it. Remember that you must relax in order to use your fingers to feel the subtle movements. (You can try this on yourself, but it's more difficult because people sometimes aren't objective enough with themselves. Do it solo, and/or try it with someone else. The fun part is watching people's eyes light up when they feel this!)

Ready for another example? Try the same exercise with your toes. Place your thumb and forefinger just below the bridge of your partner's nose, and ask your partner to do the same slow wiggle movement with the toes in one foot. You will feel the same, rolling threadlike sensation at the bridge of the nose. Some people, in fact, say the feeling is more distinct when wiggling the toes. Sometimes, varying the pressure across the nose will bring the sensation into sharper focus. Feel it now? Cool, isn't it?

You've just demonstrated that movement in one part of the body can affect the connective tissue in a distant part of the body. Moving your fingers or toes can be felt in your head! Is it any wonder that a sore shoulder can be felt as pain in the wrist or arm? That people with neck injuries experience headaches? That a tender spot in your upper arm can send a joltlike feeling of electricity shooting into your fingers?

Here's another demonstration to do on yourself. Take the thumb and fingers of your right hand and gently wrap them around the wrist of your left hand (figure 2.5A). Hold it tightly enough so your fingers and thumb make contact on the whole wrist. Now squeeze the fingers of your left hand together as if you're gripping something (figure 2.5B) and notice what you feel with your right fingers and thumb. As your fingers grip, the wrist expands. It's a simple example of the physics principle, "for every action there is an equal and opposite reaction." When you squeeze your fingers inward, your wrist expands outward. It's as if the wrist opens and braces outward to give the fingers more power. (And if you lose this stabilizing power by putting the wrist in a splint or having it cut open surgically, you lose grip in the fingers.)

Learning to feel this subtle movement now will give you a head start on understanding the concepts and techniques on which the Rossiter System stretches are based. Just as you can feel connective tissue move throughout the body, you also can stretch out the body's spiderweb system of connective tissue to make all the connected parts of the body move more fluidly and without pain. (Are you beginning to see how important this stuff is?) All you have to do is learn the right techniques, apply weight to the right areas, and stretch a certain way. The Rossiter System teaches you how to do all that.

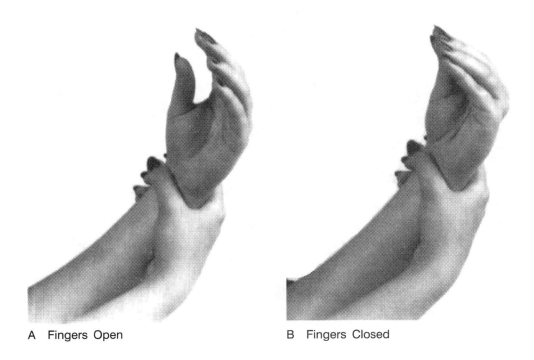

A Fingers Open   B Fingers Closed

Figure 2.5 Hand Squeeze

What Does Connective Tissue Do?

Connective tissue is critical to your existence. This incredible stuff holds everything in place—tiny cells, small muscles, little bones, big muscles, entire organs. Its most important mission is to give shape to the human body. It gives the body form and the space in which internal body parts can function normally. It holds things in place, but remember: it holds everything very gently; it wraps without squeezing.

Just as the bones and skeleton determine a person's height, just as muscles give a person strength and bulk, *connective tissue creates space within the body*. The Rossiter System simply returns lost space to the body.

Connective tissue is the soft blueprint of where everything goes. It is the guardian of the balanced body, the great equalizer, no matter how much or what kind of stress you're under. Simply put, connective tissue knows its place—and whenever possible, it returns there!

A Thought-Provoking Concept: Internal Space

Think about that. Inside your body is space. Sure, your body is filled with blood, tissue, organs, bones, and cells, but it also has space. When your hand reaches for the refrigerator-door handle, muscles, nerves, and bone expand into the space within you to make your reach happen. When you bend to pick up a child or swing a golf club, the connective tissue moves and flexes within your body to give your muscles, joints, and bones the space in which to move, bend, lift, and swing.

To consider how connective tissue works, think back to the Saran Wrap example. Suppose someone took the piece of Saran Wrap and tugged it a little. No matter where or how much it is pulled, everything—the dishes, tables, couch cushions, houses, highways, pipes, neighborhoods—would shift or move just a little bit along the entire length of wrap. The movement, connected throughout, would resemble a rippling, shifting sheet. When the pulling stopped, everything would return to its original place. Now imagine that every two feet along this wrap, someone's hand is slightly twisting this immense sheet of connective tissue. This twisting isn't at one spot, it's along the entire length of this huge wrap. The twisting will be noticed first by the dishes, later by the furniture, then by the houses, and eventually by everything else. Nobody will notice when a few dishes clink, but by the time the furniture starts moving, it will be noticeable. And when the houses start shifting, the entire system will notice the change.

That's the magnitude of connective tissue—it creates space for just about everything inside your body to happen and move, and as its name says, it's all connected, from one end to the other.

Inside the space provided by connective tissue, your body is incredibly busy. Blood, water, nutrients, and key cells circulate constantly. They deliver food, energy, nerve impulses, and messages from one part of the body to another. Glands and organs secrete special chemicals that govern reactions, behaviors, feelings, responses, and pain. Muscles and bones move, reach, bend, lift, and work. And all this takes place inside a giant connective tissue wrap.

Whatever happens to your body, inside and out, can be good or bad. Life is filled with beneficial and destructive stresses. Softball can be a good stress because it's fun and a healthy form of exercise. But sliding into second base can be a bad stress because it has the potential to sprain an ankle or cause trauma to the body's sensitive tissue.

Your body is in trouble when the tugs and pulls to connective tissue turn serious and overwhelming. Just like with the hands twisting the neighborhood sheet of Saran Wrap, the bigger the pull, the worse the entire system gets.

Pain: Your Body's Warning System

When connective tissue is overworked or injured—when the tugging is too intense or lasts too long—the body's built-in mechanism will signal something is wrong. That signal is pain. Pain is your body's way of telling you something is out of kilter. "I hurt!" it says. "Fix me!"

Maybe you feel a twinge or tingling for days on end. Maybe you have a wrenching pain in your back after lifting a heavy object improperly. Maybe your shoulder is achy after throwing a football for three hours with the kids in the backyard. Each trauma, large or small, affects everything else. When one area is pulled too tightly or worked too hard, the rest of the system is affected.

Most people associate their pain with a specific part of the body, but each part is connected with every other part. It's a systemwide phenomenon, which is a fairly different way of thinking about pain in today's world.

Here's a critical point for understanding the Rossiter System: Every human body endures a normal amount of daily wear and tear. But when connective tissue becomes stressed, it shortens and thickens, and it does so every day, depending on the kinds of activities you do.

Usually, a good night's sleep and sufficiently healthy lifestyle help the connective tissue return to normal the next day. But when connective tissue can't bounce back on a one-day turnaround, it continues to shorten and thicken, not just at the place it is overworked or stressed, but everywhere. Think of the Saran Wrap shrinking tightly around everything inside it. It squeezes and compacts valuable space and refuses to give it up. For you, it's like one big body cramp. Critical body parts cannot move fluidly. Individual cells can become damaged if they're restricted long enough. When the cramped area becomes large enough to be noticed, you experience pain.

When connective tissue tightens and thickens in that kind of scenario, you'll experience very definite sensations: tight muscles, tingling, soreness, loss of strength, buzzing, aching, throbbing, numbness, and pain. These are the major symptoms of repetitive stress injuries. In fact, all repetitive stress injuries are directly linked to a loss of space in the body.

Trauma to connective tissue comes in many forms, but one of the most destructive is *repetitive motion* (also referred to as *repetitive stress*)—repeating a movement over and over. It usually starts out as tension from working too hard or too intensely, from repeating the same movement nonstop, or from performing the same task for long periods. This tension will evolve into a lingering soreness until a particular area of your body is tight or hard all the time. This sensation is common among typists, computer and keyboard operators, slaughterhouse workers, scanner/checkout clerks, and assembly-line workers. People who prop babies on one hip for long periods know this sensation, too. So do people who exercise a lot.

Most people who experience problems like carpal tunnel syndrome or constant shoulder pain say they quit moving that particular part of the body because it hurts so much. It tingles at night. It feels numb. It aches twenty-four hours a day. Every movement produces soreness or tightness. Why? Their bodies have lost the space or range of motion necessary to maintain healthy, pain-free tissue.

Under ideal circumstances, people doing normal activities shouldn't hurt. But whenever people overuse a part of the body, the body always will respond with pain. It has to. It was designed to tell you when things aren't right.

If tension continues over a long time, or if the tension increases, the connective tissue becomes traumatized. That's why your shoulders ache after raking leaves or gardening. It's why elbows hurt after two-hour tennis matches. It's why backs hurt from carrying babies or lugging bags of groceries. The tight areas can linger or carry over into other aspects of life. Your arms might hurt from working at a computer all day, but the soreness also limits what you can do at home.

The most noticeable pains or aches will be felt at the spot where a trauma or an injury occurred, such as the ankle that jams into second base on a slide or the wrists that stay in one position for hours while typing. That specific area will become traumatized by lack of space. Its connective tissue will tighten and shorten the most. It will hurt the most.

At first, this lack of space shields the body from activity—it forces people to limp or ease up or not do something so strenuously for a time. But repeated movement in an area that's already straining and hurting becomes an ongoing trauma that gets replayed like a bad B movie. That, in essence, is a repetitive motion injury. It means a specific area's connective tissue continues to shrink and shorten because of a lack of food, poor or restricted movement, or both. And if connective tissue in a specific spot is negatively affected, connective tissue elsewhere will suffer by virtue of its connection. When people compensate for pain, it makes the entire pain situation even more complex because so many body parts, movements and habits are involved.

Let's say a repetitive motion injury starts out as a sore ankle or wrist. Usually, it just feels sore. But continue to overwork that ankle or wrist, continue to feed it more trauma or stress, and pain will eventually develop. It may be a buzzing sensation, a throbbing, or a dull morning ache in the hands, similar to arthritis. The pain of repetitive movement is slow to accumulate, but once it arrives, it seems as if it will never go away.

Once an area hurts, you might try to avoid the pain by keeping it still or restricting its movement. You may try to move around the pain by compensating for it, but compensations aren't natural. They can actually start secondary repetitive motion injuries that cause even more problems and pain over time. You might soon forget about the first pain, because the second pain now hurts even more. In fact, you might not even remember the first one.

Maybe you start doing a different job at work. Maybe you build a deck or paint a house in a single weekend. Maybe you're working more hours, using new tools, or moving a different way. Any and all of these changes can upset what's normal and balanced for your body. Your body can change and adapt without pain—to a point. But when the body can't keep up with the change and the amount of muscle tension and stress, it begins to hurt. And what used to hurt just a little now feels as if a tank plowed into you.

Acid on Your Muscles: No Wonder You're in Pain!

When muscles are forced to work beyond their limit, they produce lactic acid. It's a waste product, like garbage. It's cellular poop. It stinks. It's gross. The body wants to get rid of it. Think of it as pure lemon juice dripped onto an open cut. Does that make you want to beg for more or pucker? Pucker it is.

If that lactic acid stays near the muscle, it has to stick to something. Guess what? Connective tissue is the nearest thing, so lactic acid glues itself to connective tissue, which does exactly what your mouth does when it sips pure, sour lemon juice. It tightens. It thickens. It puckers. As more lactic acid builds up, the area tightens even more—individual cells, tiny strands of muscle fibers, entire lengths of connective tissue enclosing entire muscle groups—they all tighten and thicken. Keep in mind, this tightening is happening while the muscles and connective tissue still need a constant supply of food, nutrients, and water, so they're working extra hard even while they're stressed, puckered, and tight.

Normally, the overproduction of lactic acid is taken care of by a good night's sleep. But any job or activity that you do over and over will continue to fuel the production of lactic acid far beyond the body's ability to get rid of it. Connective tissue continues to tighten and shorten, yet muscles are forced to keep working. The result is pain.

How the Rossiter System Stretches Work on Connective Tissue

Over time, muscles and bones inside the connective tissue wrapping feel the strain of repetitive motion. What starts as a twinge evolves into a knot. That knot becomes a really sore knot, which evolves into an entire achy muscle with a sore knot. This in turn will produce a joint that seems stiff and difficult to move which produces a difficult-to-lift arm or shoulder that aches and feels locked and knotted, which in turn . . .

Get the picture? It's all one big, interconnected system.

Let's go back to the idea that connective tissue is a long rope. When a rope is slowly twisted and tightened, it eventually kinks and pops into a knot (figure 2.6). That knot isn't necessarily the trouble spot along the rope. It just happens to be the weakest link, the area that tightens and pops first. If the knot isn't unknotted, it will get bigger. If it is left untouched while the twisting continues, the tension and tightness will spread further up and down the rope. Then other knots at other weak links will pop out and grow. As these tensions grow, the joints between the areas in strain begin to ache and movement becomes much more difficult.

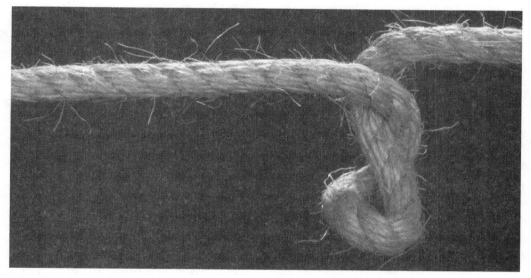

Figure 2.6   Twisted Rope

In the body, those knots occur in the connective tissue and muscles. Knots are where you'll most likely feel the pain, but the structural problem exists along the entire length of connective tissue where the pain is most noticeable. The knot may not be painful, but a nearby joint will be. The body parts most affected by knots or cramped tissue usually will be the joints or connective tissue sheaths surrounding the muscles. When everything shortens and tightens, joints are compacted and squeezed. The space between the bones lessens. Bones begin to rub against other bones.

Eventually, if the knot isn't untied, other joints, muscles, and places along that system will hurt, too. Pain might start in a wrist, for example, but soon the elbow will ache, and then a shoulder will hurt, and then headaches and neck pain will set in.

The Rossiter techniques effectively relieve pain because they stretch out entire bands of connective tissue. In essence, they untwist the entire rope and unkink all the knots. These stretches, usually by themselves, get rid of pain and restore fluid, pain-free motion to entire areas of the body.

What helps the techniques work? Connective tissue is made of different components, but two of the key fibers in the tissue are plastin and elastin. As their names indicate, they possess attributes of two everyday materials: plastic and elastic. Both can be shaped by heat and pressure. Quite simply, they can be molded. Elastin, for example, is a yellow protein that allows elastic fibers in your connective tissue to stretch up to one-and-a-half times their normal length.

Plastic fibers hold a given shape. But plastin that's been bent out of shape from stress can be remolded to its original state. How? By applying weight and movement, a combination that allows the shape of the plastic to return to normal. The Rossiter stretches are normal body movements done under weight.

When the foot is used during the Rossiter workouts, the physical foot-to-skin contact warms the underlying muscle and connective tissue, allowing it to stretch more easily (it's similar to kneading a ball of Silly Putty for a few minutes to warm it up and make it more pliable). While that is happening, you are stretching your own connective tissue, chasing out the pain by unkinking the knots and restoring tissue to its normal shape and space.

Use Rossiter as a Maintenance Program

Is the relief permanent? No. Why not? Because you still have to move, live, and work. And tomorrow, you may have to work harder, longer, or differently than you did today. The everyday tasks of lifting, carrying, driving, and playing a favorite sport can cause pain and discomfort. At work, perhaps you'll start a new task or work overtime. Maybe you'll be reassigned to a job that stresses a new part of your body. Even the most perfectly designed workstation can still cause aches and pains if the movement that's required is relentless and repetitive. The Rossiter System helps you identify any new aches and pains and get rid of them when they develop, no matter what kind of activity you do.

Chapter 3

The Four Constants of the Rossiter System

Everywhere in nature, things happen no matter how much you try to understand or whether you believe. The sun comes up each morning. Rain is always water. Stars appear in the sky. Each day that you put your feet on the ground, gravity awaits you. You don't have to smell, see, hear, or touch any of these things or phenomena. They are principles, givens, constants. They happen.

The Rossiter System is built on constants. This chapter lays out the first four. (Other constants will be explained in later chapters about back stretches.) These constants are every bit as dependable and ever-present as gravity. Our lives, in fact, depend on them.

How did these four constants evolve? Fairly early on, as part of my Rolfing practice and in the development of these techniques, I realized I needed a way to explain certain concepts to people. In my private practice, I had plenty of time to explain and talk to clients. But when I got in front of a crowd, folks acted as if I was speaking Greek. I was unable to communicate meaningfully. Perhaps I started out with a haughty attitude ("I know more than you do and want to keep it that way"). I spoke of paradigms and muscle-interaction theories and such. In retrospect, I fell prey to the approach known as "I don't know any more than you but I'll try to impress you with big words that will scare you, and you will bow in greater respect for someone as smart as I am." (The shortened version of that is "I use big words, therefore I impress.") See why I lost my audiences?

Over time, I came to my common senses. I began simplifying the core program to make it more user-friendly. I got rid of useless and complicated quasi-medical phrases that didn't hold anyone's attention. I began searching for basic concepts that people could understand and remember. I tried to remove the confusion factor.

Nature can be incredibly complex, but it doesn't have to create misery or misunderstanding. Sometimes, the simplest answers are the best answers. To that end, these four constants are at the heart of the Rossiter program.

Communication: The First Constant

The body always wants to tell you what's happening. In part, the body is designed as a feedback system to stop you from doing things that are harmful. Part of the body's job is to let you know when it's in pain. When you touch a hot iron, for example, your body jerks your finger back to prevent a burn.

When connective tissue is injured, overworked, or traumatized, it shortens. And when connective tissue shortens, the body loses its ability to communicate effectively. Nerves cannot talk optimally to the muscles, and muscles cannot talk to the greater nerve network that includes the brain.

Messages going to and coming from the brain are short-circuited, and this message breakdown happens along the entire length of connective tissue, not just where the tissue hurts.

Even though you may sense pain only in one area, or in one area more than others, entire lengths of connective tissue are actually sensing pain and feeling trauma. This is the single most important concept about connective tissue. Nerves run through connective tissue everywhere. All muscles lie within connective tissue. When muscles are restricted in movement, nerve impulses also are restricted in their ability to send messages. Remember that: these stretches are not site-specific, they are specific to entire *areas* of connective tissue. For any positive change to occur, a critical mass of connective tissue must be worked and stretched. Without addressing that critical mass, trauma and pain will reinstate themselves, because the pattern of pain, like an intricate mosaic pattern, is still in place. As long as the pattern remains embedded in the tissue, the trauma and pain will stay. The Rossiter System breaks up trauma patterns in an entire area, not just in the place of pain. All the tissues are returned to their normal, natural function.

Pain is information. It is communication. You must understand the signals your body is sending you before you can get rid of the unwanted information, or pain. By using Rossiter techniques to stretch out connective tissue to its full length, you restore the body's ability to tell you how it feels. You reactivate the body's natural communication system so it can tell you if it hurts. Your body also can tell you when it feels better. Your mission: Pay attention to what your body is telling you.

Food: The Second Constant

All tissue in the body needs a constant source of food—nutrients and oxygen. When muscles, nerves, tissues, and bones are squeezed into space that's too tight, they cannot get the proper amount of food they need. Whatever nutrients do reach the cramped tissue, they cannot be metabolized properly, which means they can't be turned into real energy. Moreover, space-starved tissue has waste products—cellular poop, as I like to call it—that it needs to get rid of.

The Rossiter stretches return to the body's tissue enough space to receive appropriate amounts of enriching nutrients and oxygen. The key word here is *appropriate*. Tight connective tissue can continue to function with an *adequate* supply of nutrients. But adequate isn't enough. Adequate means just that— enough to live. Tissue needs an appropriate amount of nutrition because it allows the tissue to remain healthy, vibrant, nourished, free of waste, and able to repair and perform freely everywhere and without restriction.

The Rossiter System replenishes the body's food supply and helps the body reach a working accord with its waste management system. Just as entire bodies crave food and want poop gone, individual cells need nourishment and a way to remove waste.

Movement: The Third Constant

Proper movement is critical for maintaining healthy tissue. If a person cannot move an area of the body the way it is designed to move, the area will deteriorate. Like a dog stuck in a doghouse, it will soon sit down and quit moving. It will weaken and shrink. Muscles are made for moving. If they cannot move, or if they cannot perform tasks, they deteriorate, weaken, shrink, and become nonfunctional.

The Rossiter stretches return the body's connective tissue to normal, allowing all tissues, organs, and body parts to move and function as they're supposed to.

Space: The Fourth Constant

Space is the crucial constant. Without space, the first three constants don't work. Everything in the body revolves around the practical idea of appropriate space. When the body and its tissues don't have enough space to move and function properly, tissue responds—it communicates—through stiffness, numbness, swelling, or pain. These pain-laden symptoms remain until the body's space requirements are satisfied.

The Rossiter stretches elongate connective tissue and return to your body the amount of space it needs to move fluidly, freely, and without pain.

Just as there are appropriate and adequate amounts of nutrients and oxygen, there are appropriate and adequate amounts of space. *Adequate* means enough space to live. A human example: a mother, father, and five kids in a two-bedroom apartment. Such a situation would involve a lot of discomfort. It would be possible, but not ideal. (Personally, I would go loony.) It's not fun and it's not a good idea. It's simply adequate.

Appropriate space is the space your body was designed to have. It's a family of seven in a four-bedroom house with two-and-a-half baths. It feels good. It feels free. It is pain-free because nothing is cramped. There are no cold spots or cramped areas. Everything feels as if it has enough space to do everything it wants. Happy tissue creates a happy person.

Every bodily function depends on this space. Space also is a critical factor in your immune system's responses. Your body is designed to act quickly and efficiently to battle ill health. Every stress on the body's appropriate space—every unfed cell, every area cramped in its ability to move—weakens your ability to ward off disease. The more restricted the body's connective tissue system, the greater the body's risk for disease, infection, and illness. Conversely, the more fluid and mobile the body is, the better able it is to remain healthy and vibrant.

Pay Heed to the Constants

These are the constants. They are the most basic of thoughts you can have regarding your body. Communication, food, and movement are absolutely basic to life. The body's need for space is evident inside and outside your body, whether it's space needed by connective tissue or space to fit inside clothes, shoes, cars, and beds. You can move, dance, play, and work inside a full-length body suit that's two sizes two small, but you certainly won't be comfortable, happy, or productive.

Likewise, violating the constants carries negative consequences. Look around you for examples. A potted plant that doesn't have enough room for its root system to soak up nutrients soon shrinks, turns brown, wilts, withers, and dies. A garden plot overrun with garbage and toxic waste becomes a non-thriving wasteland, a place where nothing grows or matures. Leave a dog in a cage for too long and the Humane Society will be at your door with warrants and questions. Why would you do to your body what you wouldn't do to a dog?

Chapter 4

The Power of Partner Stretches

There's something you should understand before you start doing these techniques: they require two people. These stretches will always involve

1. A person who needs relief from pain, tightness, tingling, soreness, numbness, or aches in the arms, hand, fingers, shoulders, neck, elbow, wrist, or back.

2. A second person who understands how to stretch out connective tissue. (Don't panic, it's easy.)

You will pair off and work together to help each other out of pain. Think of it this way: there is no finer computer than the human mind, no finer sense than the sensitivity of human touch, and no quicker feedback than the verbal messages one person gives to another.

The Person-in-Charge (PIC) and the Coach: The Heart of This Team Approach to Pain Relief

Throughout this book, you'll see references to the two people involved in the stretches: The person-in-charge (PIC) and the coach.

The *PIC* is the person in pain. You are in charge of your pain. You are its boss. Only you can work it out of your body. Usually, the PIC lies on the floor on a mat while the coach stands above. For these stretches to work, the PIC must work hard and consciously seek out and remove the pain by stretching. That may sound simple-minded, but it is the essence of the entire program.

The *coach* is the trainer, the facilitator, the person helping the PIC get out of pain. Typically, the coach stands above the PIC and uses his or her foot to apply weight at various areas on the PIC's body while the PIC performs a series of stretches. The coach supplies a steady, reassuring stream of tips, instructions, advice, and encouragement.

Got it? PIC and coach. You're a team. The PIC is in charge. The coach is there to help, encourage, goad, nudge, direct, and high-five. Think of the Rossiter System as a way for anybody to help anybody else out of pain. It's that simple. Anybody can learn these techniques. Even eight-year-olds have learned them. They are done as a series, not as individual or site-specific stretches. That's why this approach is called the Rossiter *System*—it's an entire system or series of stretching techniques, and that's where its effectiveness lies.

Once you learn the techniques, the two of you—you and a co-worker, friend, spouse, partner, child—can use them regularly. Think of this as a maintenance program for the human body, the same way you regularly change a car's oil or service a furnace. Just use the Rossiter stretches more frequently (and when you feel better, tell your friends).

You can choose how you use the stretches, too—either when you need them or as a maintenance program.

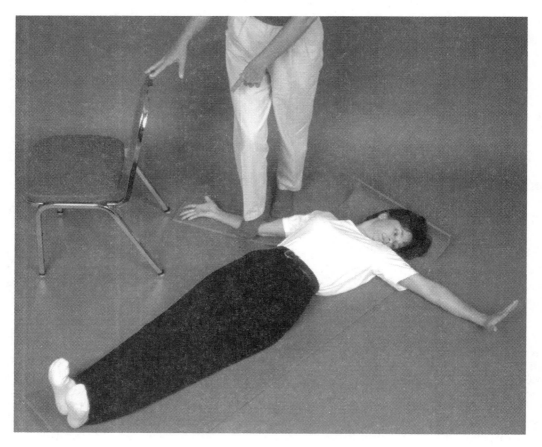

Figure 4.1   The Team

How the Foot Figures into the Rossiter Stretches

If you think these stretches look a little strange the first time you see them, you're absolutely right. After all, it's not everyday you see someone standing on someone else while they exercise or stretch out! But there are important reasons the Rossiter System uses the foot to apply weight during the stretches.

Adding weight with the foot at specific areas on muscles helps untwist and smooth out large, measured, pre-defined lengths of connective tissue until all the connective tissue is flexible and loose again. It's like smoothing out a rope that's been twisted so tight it's become knotted. When a significant part of the rope is untwisted, those tight, bulging knots pop out of place and loosen. Eventually, the whole rope relaxes.

If you know where and how to stretch critical parts of your body's connective tissue, you can get rid of pain. The Rossiter System stretches those critical parts. When your connective tissue is flexible again, you recapture the internal space your body needs to move effortlessly and without pain or tension.

Here are some other good reasons to use the foot:

▸ The bottom of the foot is smooth and can distribute weight evenly on the arm or leg.

▸ A foot works better than a hand. Pressing your hand against another person's body can create pain in your hand or wrist. There's no reason for someone to become sore while getting someone else out of pain. (When I first started teaching these techniques in public seminars, in fact, I used to advise people to use their hands to apply weight to their partners. The flaw with that approach was that many people sought out my seminars because they wanted to get rid of severe hand and wrist pain.

When they paired off to learn the stretches and were told to press on each other with their hands, those doing the pushing developed more pain, not less. Even though they were getting temporary relief from the techniques, the more they pushed on other people while doing the techniques, the more their own hands and wrists hurt. Eventually, I began advising those people to use the foot to apply weight. It worked so well that all the techniques were revised to rely on the foot as the source of weight.)

▸ It's easier to apply and accept weight from a foot. If you push on another person with a hand, he or she will instinctively push back or withdraw, which will prevent you from getting into the area that is alive with pain. If you push on a touchy, sore, or painful area, the person most likely will be anxious and will not allow you to press to the level needed to get rid of the pain. Perhaps the person will make you stop altogether.

▸ The warmth from your foot makes the underlying connective tissue a little more pliable and able to stretch.

The best and most profound change depends on the amount of connective tissue that you change. A specific spot may be the source of your immediate achiness (your wrist, for example), but pain is actually coming from a larger area, an extensive web of interacting muscles, bones, nerves, and blood vessels (those involving your wrist, arms, shoulders, and neck). They are all surrounded and interwoven with connective tissue—the very stuff to which these stretches are geared. If you loosen the surrounding connective tissue, all the surrounding cells feel better.

After you've done this series of stretches several times, the positive changes occur more rapidly because you've already worked out years of built-up stress that your body is harboring. The pain or tightness that remains may be only weeks or months worth of significant stress. Once you practice these stretches regularly, it's easier to get rid of pain—and the process is a lot less painful. People who use the Rossiter System regularly are accustomed to being pain-free. In fact, they expect it.

If you aren't quite comfortable with the thought of someone else's big, smelly foot on your body, think about this: Wouldn't you prefer a stinky foot to surgery, shots, or pills? Make sure the coach wears clean socks every time and you should be fine. Stay away from nylons and people who don't wear socks with leather shoes.

Why Weight?

There's a difference between *weight* and *pressuring* or *pushing*. Pressing and pushing imply that it's necessary to use sheer strength to get results. Weight is not necessarily invasive. Muscling someone is. If you push someone, she'll tighten and push back. If you lean against someone, he will either move or shift his weight to accommodate yours.

But when you apply weight with your foot, there's no sudden change in the other body's musculature. Weight from a foot doesn't feel as if someone is trying to invade a scary area. It feels more right, more natural. Resistance from a foot is minimal. If weight is added slowly enough, the person receiving it will allow it to happen, even if it may be slightly painful or uncomfortable.

Weight from the foot, applied at specific areas on the body, is what makes these stretches so effective. Notice I used the term *specific areas*. To get any area of connective tissue to unwind, it's necessary to stretch a critical mass of connective tissue. That's why it's important to use the whole system of Rossiter techniques, not pick and choose one or two. Using the entire system of stretches ensures that the right problem is being addressed with the proper solution.

How Much Weight Is Enough?

Until you've done these stretches a few times, you'll no doubt wonder if the coach's foot is adding enough weight to be effective. The key to the concept of weight is cooperation between the coach and the PIC. Each stretch involves the PIC's soft tissue and muscle under the coach's foot and five powerful concepts. If you both understand your responsibilities during a workout, you'll produce excellent results.

Weight is the first concept. Weight is simple. The coach must apply enough weight with his or her foot to make a difference in the stretch. How much is enough?

If you're the PIC and you feel as if your eyes are about to pop out of your head when your coach steps on or adds weight to you, that's enough. Conversely, Coach, if your PIC's eyes look as if they're about to pop, stop adding weight at that point. At peak moments like this, you'll both want to communicate about what's tolerable and what's not. Remember, the eyes tell it all, so keep your eyes open and try to work with a friend. Learning how much weight is enough is what makes this system work. It will take a few days for the coach to get a good feel of how much weight to add and for the PIC to figure out how much weight can be handled.

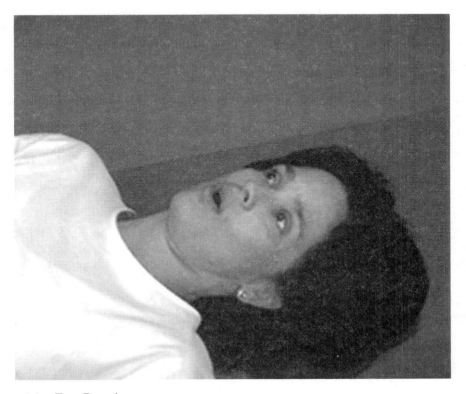

Figure 4.2 Eye Popping

Essentials of the Partner System

Appropriate Weight

Let me make it clear these stretches are not for wimps. The path of pain is sometimes hidden and stored—more than you know—throughout your body. These techniques work because they allow you to go into your body, hunt for pain, find it, and stretch it out. Wimps tell you how bad their pain is, how nobody can do anything for it, how they've visited an endless stream of doctors and chiropractors and physical therapists to no avail, how painkillers no longer work, and how surgery is the next step. In my experience, most "wimps" have been duped to believe someone else has the solution to their pain.

In the Rossiter System, the only person in charge of pain is the PIC—and that's you. When the coach adds weight to your arm or shoulder during a stretch, there is no room for wimpiness. The addition of weight should feel more than uncomfortable. It should make you wish you were somewhere else. It might bring you close to tears. When the coach sees those kinds of signs, it's enough weight. That's effective weight. (The instructions for the individual stretches include specific tips for avoiding injury and adjusting weight.)

The weight is delivered slowly and smoothly by the coach. And AFTER the weight is added, then the real work of the stretch begins!

Stretching Limits

Stretching is the Great Indicator of how willing the PIC is to get rid of pain. The stretch is commitment. The more profound the stretch, the better the results. A seemingly small detail (figure 4.3), such as how far apart the fingers are stretched, can make a great difference in the effectiveness of the carpal tunnel techniques. The palm should be whitish and fingers should be stretching and reaching as far as they can. If all you accomplish is a so-so hand stretch, you'll get so-so results. Pay attention to details, and always stretch to capacity.

No one gets positive results from Rossiter stretches except the person willing to go the length to make them work. It is control that you, and only you, have. You can fake it to someone else, you can swear you're working hard when you're really not, or you can swear the stretches aren't really working for you—and you'll be right. They won't work because you haven't put forth the effort to get good results. It's easy to cheat when you stretch, but you're the one who suffers. And as the coach gets better at coaching, you won't be able to get away with as much cheating. The coach will know when you're cheating, and if he or she is truly a friend, will call you on it.

Stretching is simple, but it's not easy. It's simply hard work.

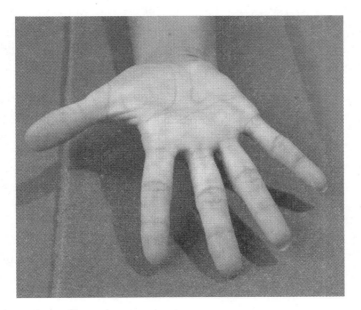

Figure 4.3   Stretch to Capacity

Location! Location! Location!

Location is the coach's responsibility. That means the coach must know where to add weight and make sure the PIC's body is Locked properly for each stretch to work. The Locks and locations are described in chapter 8 and in the instructions for each stretch.

Proper Technique

Technique means the coach must know the proper order and movements required during each stretch. It also means making sure the PIC returns to a neutral position—relaxed, hands down at sides, breathing—after each stretch. Most importantly, it means not letting the PIC cheat or wimp out during the workout. For example, if the PIC does not return the hands to the sides after each stretch, the next repetition of the technique doesn't integrate itself into the rest of the body. Integration produces lasting results, and the coach who insists on sticking to the details is the best coach.

It's All in the Details

Details means what it says. Details. The little bits of information and reminders that accompany each stretch, even though they may seem insignificant or inconsequential, are critical. If the details are ignored or only partially enforced, the whole system of stretches suffers and the results are weak or not as effective as they should be. In essence, the whole Rossiter System becomes a shell of the Rossiter System when the details slide. If you're the coach and you let someone get by or cheat because it's your buddy, spouse, friend, or boss, the techniques become ineffective and weak. Without watching the details, a PIC will be inclined to cheat more. As a coach, continually razz your PIC to stick with the details. Let the PIC know you're the coach—you're there to make sure the PIC works hard and not waste time. To bone up on the details, read and re-read chapter 9 on crosschecks before you start your workouts.

Remember, these stretches produce powerful results if the PIC and coach work as a team and understand his or her own and each other's roles and goals. Go team!

Chapter 5

Why Traditional Methods Don't Work: The Lowdown on Drugs, Shots, Splints, and Surgery

An unfortunate thing has happened to the human body: it has become "medicalized." Many people have not experienced the body's innate power to heal itself, given the right tools and information. Maybe no one ever told them such power exists. The medical establishment won't tell them, because it's in the industry's best interest to grow, and in order to grow, it must continue to manage things medically. If there's no money to be made in certain approaches to health and prevention, the medical system typically doesn't offer them.

Medical Options (and Why They Don't Work)

With carpal tunnel syndrome and other bodily aches and pains, the solutions offered by traditional medicine often aren't solutions at all. They're quick fixes. They're masks. They're bait-and-switch approaches that prevent the body from healing itself. Sometimes, they have damaging side effects. But they're all for sale!

Moreover, all current forms of medical intervention ignore one basic tenet: *Pain is information.* Pain can be dealt with using simple techniques like the Rossiter stretches. Pain relief doesn't require sense-numbing pills or potentially dangerous shots or invasive surgery.

Chronic pain that's embedded in your body is a structural problem. It is not caused by a lack of drugs in your system. It is not an automatic reason to perform surgery. (A chiropractor friend of mine figures most doctors must look at the human body and pronounce it "deficient in Tylenol and possessing a few too many organs.") Body pain is usually an interplay of the body's structures—its bones, muscles, joints, and connective tissues. The body hurts because that system has been misused, overused, or abused. It makes sense that a structural problem calls for a structural solution. The Rossiter System fixes the body's structural system by restoring its natural functions, abilities, and space.

Let's look at why today's medical options don't work.

Option 1: Painkillers and Pills

When tissue is damaged, it naturally swells. That's the body's way of trying to heal itself. Swelling sends a message that something is injured or wrong. It's also the body's way of sending more blood to an injured area to nourish and bathe it with extra nutrients, deliver oxygen, and give it added capability to carry away waste products. Often, swelling immobilizes an injured area to prevent further damage.

Non-steroidal anti-inflammatories (NSAIDs) are usually prescribed or suggested to stop the swelling and inflammation. As the name suggests, NSAIDs are not steroids; they're drug compounds that reduce the swelling reaction that the body naturally sets in motion. These kinds of drugs (prescription and over-the-counter) include Advil, Nuprin, Motrin, Excedrin, Naprosyn, Naproxen, Anaprox, and the like (the active ingredient is usually acetaminophen or ibuprofen).

Sometimes, muscle relaxants are prescribed for muscle sprains, backaches, or generalized aches, pains, and strains. These include prescription drugs such as Flexeril, Robaxin, Norflex, Soma, and the generic drug baclofen.

Essentially, NSAIDs and other painkilling, anti-swelling drugs stop the body's natural healing response. Because they're synthetic, the body isn't sure what to do with them. These unnatural chemicals interfere with the body's normal channels of information and pain sensation. The information becomes bleary and fuzzy. As a result, the senses become masked or diluted—even with drugs like Tylenol. Because pill-takers can't feel their pain, they continue using and overusing the injured area, literally adding insult to injury.

In a few days, the body figures out the pill's chemical combination and disarms the drug. Then what happens? The pain returns, and the drug is no longer effective. Usually, people switch to different or more powerful drugs (or take two pills instead of one, and then three instead of two). The pain cycle starts again. Permanent pain relief, unfortunately, never arrives.

It's important to understand that your body disarms drugs for a reason: it has to tell you it's in pain. Your body has to alert you that pain remains and that you need to do something constructive to fix the source of the problem.

In addition, NSAIDs and other drugs have side effects. Just read any label. They slow down essential blood to the injured area, causing tissue to deteriorate further (even though you may not feel it). They can cause dizziness, nausea, stomach pain, ulcers, and headaches. Muscle relaxants decrease the sensitivity of injured muscle or tissue, slow the muscle's natural responses, and make people not really care whether they hurt. Side effects of muscle relaxants include drowsiness, dizziness, confusion, nausea, anorexia, or fatigue. People taking these kinds of drugs are often a danger to themselves and their colleagues.

Here's how serious drug side effects can be: A University of Toronto study in the *Journal of the American Medical Association* (Lazarou 1998) found that "adverse reactions'" to prescription drugs in 1994 killed 106,000 Americans in hospitals and injured another 2.2 million. Those numbers do not take into account people who suffered negative side effects from drugs outside of hospital settings. Those statistics make prescription-drug side effects the sixth-leading cause of death in the United States, behind heart disease, cancer, stroke, lung disease, and accidents. According to the study, prescription drugs kill more people a year than pneumonia and diabetes. Now, do you want to risk taking more pills?

Pills violate the first constant discussed in chapter 3—communication. Your body needs to communicate within itself. Communication is a vital function. Pills violate this most necessary bodily function by shutting down, muzzling, or interfering with the body's internal signals.

It's interesting to note here that the medical profession keeps changing the words, terms, and phrases it uses to describe its treatments. Pills are now "oral medications." "Medicines" are now "medications." Sounds better, more official, doesn't it? Pills are still pills; drugs are still drugs, no matter what they're called.

Option 2: Splints

How many times have you seen computer operators or checkout clerks working with splints or braces on their wrists? While they may stabilize an area that's hurting or overworked, splints possess a major logical flaw. By restricting movement to a particular area of the body, they tax and overwork nearby muscles, bones, and tissues, sending the injury somewhere else. (For example, a few weeks after a splint is applied to a wrist, pain can begin to spread to the fingers, elbow, or shoulder.)

Splints also restrict blood flow. They're usually placed on a wrist or arm so tightly that they leave red marks on the skin when they're removed. Remember how connective tissue creates space in the body? When connective tissue is squeezed or constricted, space is lost. Remember how blood is important to feed and nourish muscles and tissues? When splints squeeze an injured area, the body's natural healing process is blocked.

Decreasing blood flow, restricting movement, and reducing the amount of space available to tissue usually means the return of a major symptom: numbness. Unfortunately, people with carpal tunnel syndrome or wrist pain see numbness as a necessary evil, thinking, "Well, at least it doesn't hurt anymore." What they should be asking is, "Is it getting well? Is it improving? Is it healing so that eventually the splint can come off?"

The answer to those questions is a simple "no." Splints do not help injured tissue or sore joints improve. When muscles don't move, they atrophy. They stiffen, shrink, and lose their usefulness. And when that happens, another area of the body must come to the rescue and work harder, setting up a vicious cycle of overuse and more pain somewhere else.

Look at how the medical profession uses words to describe these devices. "Braces," which sounds restrictive and formidable, are now "splints." They perform the same function but with a new name that's supposedly easier on the psyche.

Option 3: Cortisone Shots

If you had a chance to peer inside a human body that's been subjected to repeated cortisone shots, you might not like what you see. "Macerated necrotic tissue" is how one neurosurgeon describes it. "Like mush." (*Macerated*, in case you're wondering, means "to waste away or to cause to waste away, to become soft or separated into constituent elements . . . as if by steeping in fluid," according to *Webster's New World Dictionary*. *Necrotic* means dead. Yuck.)

An orthopedic surgeon and sports medicine specialist describes tissue that's been subjected to too much cortisone as matted, brownish or yellow, weakened, and just plain old. Sometimes, if the cortisone isn't injected at just the right spot, tiny crystals of the drug will linger in the tissue or on the joint, like gritty pieces of irritating sand on otherwise smooth, gliding surfaces.

Is that what you want medical treatments to do to sensitive, necessary, living tissue inside your body?

Cortisone is a steroid hormone that's produced naturally by your adrenal glands. It helps your body store glucose, an energy-food source, and regulate its use of fats, salts, and blood. It also helps your body deal with stress, among other things. The synthetic form of cortisone is called prednisone. Corticosteroids are synthetic steroid drugs that act like cortisone in the body.

Doctors use cortisone/prednisone because it is a powerful drug for reducing swelling. In people with arthritis, it keeps painful, swollen joints from rubbing against each other. It's also used to treat allergies and poison ivy—both of which are reactions that involve swelling. It can be taken as a pill or injected directly into joints. Xylocaine, Lanacane, and other numbing agents are sometimes used separately or in conjunction with cortisone to numb the skin or underlying tissue before a cortisone shot is given. Think about that—getting one shot to dull an area to get another shot that kills pain. Does that make any sense?

When cortisone was first introduced in the 1940s, it was hailed as a miraculous cure for arthritis, according to *100 Drugs That Work* by Mike Oppenheim, M.D. (1994). As soon as it was adopted for widespread use among arthritis patients, however, doctors started noticing that it created more problems than it "cured."

When the drug was stopped, patients' joint pain grew worse than before treatment. Used too frequently, cortisone began wearing away and eroding the naturally smooth bone surfaces that glide against each other at joints. Nearby muscles, when subjected to cortisone shots, began to weaken, discolor, thin, and lose strength.

According to the *Mayo Clinic Health Letter*, side effects from long-term cortisone/prednisone use can include muscle weakness, swollen and puffy tissues, osteoporosis, slow wound healing, thinning of skin, elevated blood pressure, weakened immune system, and emotional distress. If you have diabetes, it can worsen the disease. Other cortisone side effects, listed in the *1998 Physicians' Desk Reference*, are glaucoma, cataracts, and a tendency for the drug to mask existing and new infections—and those are infections anywhere in the body.

Today, cortisone is not meant to be used as a long-term treatment for joint pain or muscle injuries, and ethical doctors use it only if they think it's necessary, as a last resort. Moreover, they limit how many shots they'll administer to a specific area or joint and some doctors say three to six injections is the maximum—in a life. *The Johns Hopkins Medical Handbook* (Margolis 1995), in discussing corticosteroid injections into joints for arthritis, also recommends limits: "Because more frequent use increases the risk of damage to the cartilage, these injections should only be performed once or twice a year."

When I was a practicing Rolfer, I repeatedly saw the negative effects of cortisone shots that had been given up to ten to twenty years earlier. Patients who had received cortisone shots had what looked like holes or puckers where a cortisone-injection needle had been inserted into the skin and underlying tissue. That hole or dent represents the rotting of underlying tissue. It can be seen and it can be felt by pressing on it. It sometimes felt slick or greasy under the skin. Cortisone patients say the site of the shot sometimes feels painful or numb. People often call it the "cortisone pucker."

Muscle and tissue is damaged directly more by cortisone shots than by any other medical treatment for structural problems, except for surgery, because cortisone scars tissue physically and chemically. It changes calcium and sugar levels in your body. It weakens muscle. It is corrosive and literally rots the tissue over time. (Is it any wonder the pain goes away? When there's nothing left of the tissue, there's nothing to be felt). Then something worse happens.

Once subjected to cortisone, tissue has to rebuild from scratch. It's a long process, one that may take years. Cortisone actually slows the connective tissue's ability to regenerate and heal. Sometimes, the tissue never heals, and in older people, scarring can last for life. The worst part is that when pain returns, it comes back with a vengeance. And it rarely goes away. You just have to live with it. Think of it this way: You've got dead tissue living next door to healthy tissue, rubbing sides and trying to coexist. If you were the living tissue, wouldn't you raise a storm of protest?

And back to the medicinal word games that surround this treatment. "Shots" have become "injections" because nobody likes to get shot, right?

Is it any wonder the medical field says cortisone is a last resort before surgery? I don't think it's ever a last resort. To me, a last resort is the farthest place on the map before the wilderness. It's beautiful. It's a paradise. The fishing is good, the food is excellent, and you don't ever want to leave. Does that sound like a cortisone shot? Not to me. When doctors tell you it's a last resort, think seriously about the meaning and consider other options.

Option 4: Surgery

Our bodies are not meant to be opened. Yet many people with carpal tunnel syndrome resort to surgery that cuts the transverse carpal ligament in the wrist. The surgery automatically reduces strength in the hand 20 to 30 percent. That loss is permanent, and it's why many employers don't like to hire people who have had carpal tunnel surgery (however, they can no longer discriminate because of the Americans with Disabilities Act).

Women tend to scar more easily than men, so women often lose more of their grip after surgery. People who have undergone carpal tunnel surgery often say they have "tired" hands ("I can't lift another thing" is a frequent complaint). They may experience constant or sharp hand pain. They may appear lazy or slow when their hands are in pain.

Whenever surgery is performed, a certain amount of scar tissue forms. Scar tissue is dead tissue, just liked the atrophied tissue created by cortisone shots. Scarring shortens or tightens surrounding tissue. Nearby skin and tissue feel as if they're being pulled. Movement in the immediate area feels restricted. Sometimes an elbow, wrist, finger, or hand is not able to flex or bend the way it could before surgery. Range of motion becomes narrower. Nearby tissue sometimes has the sensation of feeling cool, numb, or painful. All these are indicators of a loss of space in the tissue.

Again, pay attention to the words doctors now use when recommending cutting and severing tissue. "Surgeries" have become "procedures" or "techniques." See how much less invasive it sounds? If you're just having a procedure, goes the thinking, what's to worry about?

As with any surgery, please look at all your options and ask hard, serious questions before making a decision. Ask about benefits, drawbacks, side effects, short- and long-term results, recovery, options, and the doctor's experience and success rate with this particular kind of surgery. And don't forget to ask about being able to return to your work and hobbies. Ask to talk to other patients (of this particular surgeon) before agreeing to any kind of surgery.

Option 5: Ergonomic Evaluation, Work Reassignment, or Physical Therapy

Many offices and factories today hire ergonomics experts—people who specialize in designing environments or equipment that adapt to the human body. Ergonomics professionals often can make work more comfortable by making equipment easier to use. They might suggest or do the following:

Switch workers to different jobs, or rotate workers into different but slightly similar jobs, when one task produces pain. In reality, most jobs in factories today are very much the same. Often, they're just a slight hand movement different from other tasks. Most companies keep an injured worker on the same assembly line doing a slight variation of the original job. The only difference is that it might be farther down the line or closer to the snack machine. Rarely is there any significant change.

Use new equipment or use existing equipment differently. Both approaches will sometimes help, but this approach has limitations. I've been in many companies that have changed the entire assembly process to get rid of all their carpal tunnel problems—only to have complaints about elbow and shoulder pain, soreness, muscle aches, and injuries recur in about six months.

Often the same injuries return but in a different place on the body (for example, the repetitive motion injury is no longer at the wrist, it's at the elbow, or it's on the inside of the wrist instead of the outside of the wrist). Some companies will again change entire systems, only to have problems crop up *again*. Because of costs, companies sometimes reconfigure only the most troublesome spot(s) on the assembly line, or they try to figure out solutions only for people who complain.

Ergonomics is a critically important field, but it can never completely solve all the problems. If you're a factory worker who has to use a vibrating rivet gun hundreds of times a day, even the best ergonomically designed tool and workstation can't cut your quota or the number of times you must lift, push, and pop the rivet in place. If you're a nurse who must lean over a medical cart to hand out pills, all that leaning will eventually take its toll, no matter how well designed the cart and how conscientious you are about leaning, lifting, and bending correctly.

When carpal tunnel syndrome was first recognized as a major occupational injury, its definition was limited to the wrist. Over the past few years, repetitive stress injuries similar to carpal tunnel syndrome are increasingly occurring farther up the arm, from the hand into the elbow or shoulder. Each time the injury transfers or moves from the wrist into more critical areas of the body, it becomes harder and more expensive to fix. Unfortunately, ergonomics can never fix the problem completely. Often, it just transfers or shuttles it somewhere else.

In addition to ergonomics evaluations, workers sometimes are referred to physical therapy for exercise or occupational therapy to prepare them to return to work. Physical therapy can help, but it has limitations. Most physical therapy clients learn how to stretch muscles, not connective tissue. Most therapy concentrates on balancing muscle groups but doesn't address the underlying problem, and often the work is too localized or limited. Physical therapy's major drawback, in my opinion, is that it doesn't address the entire system of connective tissue.

The Rossiter Option

The Rossiter System provides the only true way to get rid of pain: stretch out your entire system of connective tissue, from the tip of your fingers, up through your arms, into your shoulders and neck, down into your back, and into your legs and feet. Each Rossiter workout provides an all-encompassing stretch. The more connective tissue is stretched, the better the results. A Rossiter workout also provides better long-term results, meaning the positive effects from a single stretching session last longer than the effects of other kinds of stretches. Your tissue returns to its normal state and is able to carry out its normal functions.

And here's the best thing about the Rossiter System: It has no side dangerous side effects. The Rossiter System is about getting yourself back to normal—and staying normal.

Part II

The Stretches

Chapter 6

Disclaimers, Contraindications, and Limitations

Read this before attempting any of these stretches to protect yourself from injury and to make sure you're not putting yourself or your partner at risk!

Disclaimers

This is not a treatment. The Rossiter System does not claim to treat anyone, anytime, anywhere. We do not use the term "treat" or "treatment." It is illegal in many states to use medical terminology, and we are not medical practitioners in any sense, nor do we pretend to be.

The Rossiter System is a service provided to people. It is a service based on specific knowledge. We provide techniques for people to use on themselves with the assistance of another person. This is about people empowering themselves to get rid of their own pain.

The Rossiter System has been used in several dozen American factories and offices for ten years, and it has never resulted in a lawsuit.

Contraindications

If in doubt, don't do these stretches! This is especially true if the Person-in-Charge has undergone surgery. In a work situation, a surgeon must clear injured patients or people who've had surgery before they're allowed to return to work and resume activities. Similarly, in our factory-based work, any person who has had surgery must give written consent to the coach in order to do the workouts.

Granted, things are different when you're stretching with a family member or friend, but unless consent of some kind has been given by the PIC to the coach, it is not recommended to work together. Blame is a terrible game to play. Nobody wins. Before starting the System, make sure you've read and understood the following:

▶ Never do these techniques on a broken bone.

▶ Stay off the joints when applying weight. **Never** add weight with your foot to the PIC's joint.

▶ Do not work on open wounds, rashes, sores on the skin, contagious diseases, cancers, or anything of an unusual nature. If you're in doubt, play it safe and wait until your partner has been cleared by a doctor before trying these stretches.

▶ Do not stretch an area if the PIC has received a cortisone shot in that area in the last six months. This is especially true of the back and neck.

➤ Do not stretch a PIC who has had surgery in the last six months.

➤ If the PIC has Norplant contraceptive filaments implanted under the skin of her upper arm, do not apply weight or do any stretches in that area.

➤ Do not stretch a PIC who has a pacemaker.

➤ If the PIC is using a nicotine patch to help quit smoking, do not stretch or apply weight to the area where the patch is applied (it can increase the amount of nicotine absorbed through the skin).

➤ Do not stretch a PIC who has undergone a chiropractic treatment the same day or someone who has been under a chiropractor's care less than six months.

➤ Do not stretch a woman who has breast implants.

➤ If the PIC wears splints, the PIC must give permission to remove them and try the stretches.

Precautions and Limitations

Like all programs and techniques, the Rossiter System has limitations in conjunction with certain conditions.

Cortisone Shots and Surgery

These stretches are least effective in people who have had cortisone shots or surgery, or both, to treat repetitive motion injuries, joint pain, or other musculoskeletal injuries. The cortisone-surgery combination can cause incredible tissue damage, and the damage takes a long time to erase, if at all.

If you're simply looking for another quick fix to your body's pain, this probably won't work, either. It is not a miracle, and it is not always quick. The Rossiter System stretches work because you make them work. Remember that: You do this work.

One factor makes a difference, and that is persistence. Over a long period, it's your own investment of time, hope, and persistence that will change and improve the connective tissue inside your body and get rid of your aches and pains. Sometimes, especially if other medical modalities or treatments have been used, it may take one or two years to recover even half the movement, fluidity, and range of motion you once had. Remember, your injuries happened slowly and insidiously. In most cases, they developed over months and years. It may take that long to return your body to a normal, pain-free state. When you decide you don't have the time, inclination, or desire to fix yourself, or if you decide to let a doctor or other medical professional make all the decisions for you, then you've given away the power to heal yourself.

That's why persistence is so important. Stick with this program, and it will make a positive difference in how you feel, move, live, play, and work.

Rheumatoid Arthritis

Many people with rheumatoid arthritis—a type of arthritis marked by swelling and painful joints—do not follow through with all the Rossiter techniques. They tend to give up quickly because the stretches hurt. It's especially important, however, for arthritis sufferers to perform all the techniques in a balanced manner.

If you start the stretches and give up, the pain will feel worse because the tissue is "stuck" in the middle of healing. It's temporarily opened or stretched, but when you quit, it returns to its previous state of pain. I recommend these stretches only for people who are persistent by nature.

Try this: Do the stretches on one side of your body only for the first two weeks. Start on the side that hurts least because it takes a definite commitment to go after the first pain. If you can do the "easy" side first, then you will be more likely to have the gumption to go after the difficult side later. (If you start on the most painful side, you might give up more readily.)

As you work one side, notice and compare changes. Pay attention to how much freedom of movement you have. Pay attention to how the joints and limbs on one side of your body move and feel, in comparison with the other side of your body. Chances are you'll feel the difference.

In my opinion, all arthritis is a form of shortening of the body's connective tissue. When arthritis flares up, people do nothing or they take pills. By choosing those two options, they allow further degeneration of the joints and allow the shortening of connective tissue to continue. And taking pills can cause arthritis sufferers to do things they normally wouldn't—play golf all day or overexert themselves. Then they hurt worse the next day, and fall back into a pattern of pills and inactivity.

A daily regimen of stretches throughout life will prevent arthritis in its many aching forms. Make sure the stretches are done slowly and steadily. Make sure pain is diminishing before you move out of each stretch. If you leave pain during its peak, you will need to return to it in another movement or stretch.

If you're in doubt about the Rossiter workout, do the stretches on just one side of your body for a few days and notice the difference. Compare how it feels with the unstretched side.

Cramping

Cramps can occur when you overload the muscle groups you're stretching or by overzealous tightening of the muscles near the area being stretched. Usually, people undergoing Rossiter stretches get cramps because they perform general movements or the Locking position improperly. (You'll read about Locking in chapter 8.)

Here's a tip: Let your back relax while doing these stretches! Don't Lock or reach too hard. Let the arms, legs, and heels do the bulk of the work. Your back should not tighten up. If you do get a cramp in your back, it means you were relying too heavily on your back or you were straining your arm. The remedy? Stop stretching, sit up, wait a few minutes, lie back down, and start again.

Chapter 7

What You'll Need to Do These Stretches

Here's one of the great things about the Rossiter System: you don't have to open your wallet and invest in anything special for the stretches to work. (Okay, maybe open it just a crack.) With the Rossiter partner stretches, there are no monthly fees. No long-term contracts. No operators standing by.

This is all you'll need for an effective workout:

▶ A room large enough to allow one of you to lie down

▶ A pair of clean socks for the coach

▶ A chair the coach will use for balance (A kitchen chair works fine.)

▶ This book to help you step-by-step through the series of stretches

▶ The desire and determination to get rid of your pain

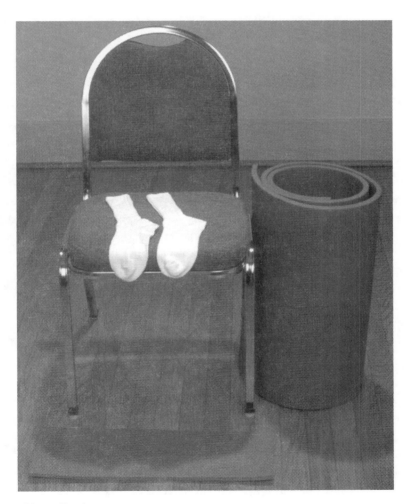

Figure 7.1 Your Tools

▸ A carpet or protective mat, such as an exercise mat or a camping mat, on the floor for the PIC (look for the dense-foam ¾-inch thick camping mats, which work much better than exercise mats.)

▸ A smaller mat or a blanket to place under the PIC's arm when working on stretches that involve the arm (it's easiest to make the smaller mat yourself. Buy a foam camping mat and cut six inches off the end. Use the main piece as the mat for the PIC to lie on and use the end piece as an arm placement mat. Or you could use a small blanket as an arm-supporting mat.)

The more you do these stretches with other people, the more you'll notice that no two human bodies are alike. In fact, bodies are vastly different. Because of these differences, you'll notice a distinct need to pad or prop up some people's body parts now and then.

When the PIC needs a pad or extra support, you'll notice immediately. The extra support will usually be necessary in three areas: knees, neck, and arms.

Neck

The neck is the most important and most critical area to support. Some people's backs are so curved that their necks also curve when they lie down, causing their heads to tilt too far back (as in figure 7.2A) to do these stretches safely. Rolling the head to the side will hurt. Vertebrae will be at an odd angle to the ground or the rest of the body. Their nostrils will point up into the air, not at their toes and feet. They may need a small (emphasis on small) pad on which to lay the head (as in figure 7.2B). This pad ensures that they can still roll the head away comfortably and safely when asked to Lock. Do not use a pad directly under the neck. Use it only to support the back of the head.

Arms/Wrists

Some bone structures are such that when a person's arm lies flat on a pad, a flippy-looking wrist pops up and hangs in the air. It's like a teeter-totter reaction: When one part goes down flat, the other pops up. What should you do?

If you decide to position the PIC to perfection by pushing the offending wrist to the floor, you may be amazed at what happens. As you push the wrist down, the shoulder rises four to six inches into the air, creating what seems to be a new human-form species. You've got two options here: Return the wrist to the air and place a pad under it, or place a pad under the PIC's uplifted shoulder and continue the stretch that way.

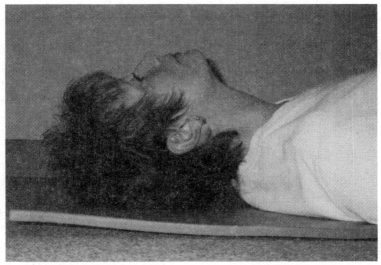

A　Bad Neck Position

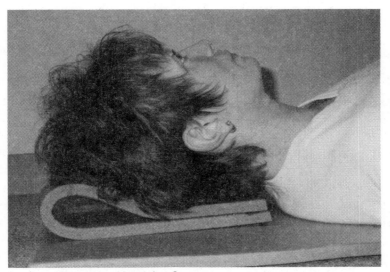

B　Pad Under the Head for Support

Figure 7.2　Neck Support

Do what each situation calls for, because this person's wrist and shoulder cannot both be on the floor at the same time. It's anatomically impossible. Accommodate your partner and his or her body type. If you're working on the forearm, let the shoulder be elevated and supported. When you're working on the shoulder, let the wrist be flippy.

Knees

For the Rossiter System stretches, knee support is needed only for the back stretches. Knees can either be bent (which is easier) or they can be propped up from underneath with some kind of pad or bolster for comfort (figure 7.3).

Some people cannot have their backs worked on because they've undergone back surgery. Those same people, however, can do the Rossiter arm stretches if they can lie on the floor. That's where padding and supporting the knees can help. The PIC needs to be as comfortable as possible during the stretches, or arm pain will continue.

Use knee supports only if they're necessary. Don't use them solely for comfort. It's more important to stretch well than it is to be perfectly comfortable. Whenever possible, have the PIC raise his or her toes while the heels are firmly planted on the mat. Only the PIC's heels should rest on the mat when doing this. The soles should be in the air. This is a modified Lock, which will be addressed in chapter 8.

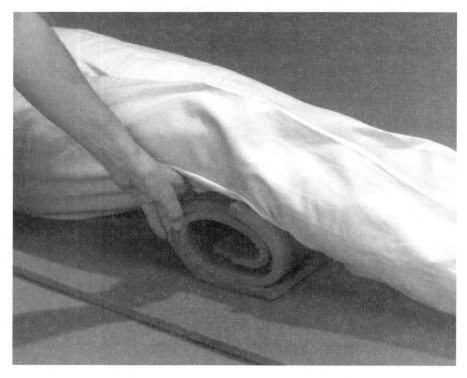

Figure 7.3   Knee Support

What to Wear?

Ideally, both coach and PIC should wear loose, comfortable clothes, but these stretches can be done anytime, anyplace in any type of clothing. Do them at work, at home, on the job, at lunch, during a break, at the gym, or at the ball field.

Chapter 8

Before You Start

Glossary

Several phrases and words show up during the stretches. Here's a brief glossary to help you remember the people and concepts involved in the Rossiter program.

Base Foot: The foot on which the coach rests and balances during the stretches.

Coach: The person who helps someone in pain stretch out. The coach typically stands up while coaching, instructing, and directing the series of stretches.

Hole in the Shoulder: The name of the last upper-body stretch and also a fleshy spot in the shoulder, below the shoulder bone and just above the armpit. Into that spot, away from bone, the coach adds weight with a heel during the actual stretch.

Locking: A position done by the Person-in-Charge (PIC) during each stretch. The PIC pulls the feet and toes toward the head, sweeps the unstretched arm along the floor with a straight elbow, palm facing out and fingers pointed at the ceiling until the arm is perpendicular to the torso, and gently rolls the head toward the shoulder.

Mr. Twister: A soothing technique done by the coach when the PIC feels stinging, buzzing, or residual pain after a stretch. It's a gentle hold and twist held for 30 seconds or more on the sore area created by the technique.

Person-in-Charge (PIC): The person in pain who is doing the stretches. Typically, the PIC lies on the floor while the coach helps and instructs while standing.

Tiny Torque: Another soothing technique done by the coach when a PIC feels stinging, buzzing, or lingering pain created by the stretch. Using the ball of the foot, the coach adds a small amount of weight and gently turns the tissue under the foot, holding it for up to 30 seconds or more on the sore body part. This technique soothes and sucks out residual pain.

Working Foot: The foot with which the coach adds weight to a PIC's body during the stretches (see chapter 4).

Locking: The Key to Effective Stretches

A guitar or violin sounds better when its strings are tautly and finely tuned. The human body works the same way, and a position called *Locking*, or *Locking Up*, gives all the Rossiter techniques the most powerful stretch available to the human body's connective tissue.

Locking powers the Rossiter techniques to perform at their best. It's a way of reaching out with the heels, the palm of the hand, and the head to make sure the body's connective tissue is stretched to its fullest capacity on one side of the body while you're executing a specific Rossiter stretch on the other side. Locking is done after the coach has applied weight with his or her foot.

Here's how to Lock when your coach tells you to. Remember, these Locking movements are done simultaneously and fluidly. Once you get the hang of it, Locking comes naturally.

1. From a relaxed position with arms at your side, sweep one arm along the floor out to the side with your elbow locked, wrist on the floor, palm facing out and fingers pointing toward the ceiling, as if you're gesturing to stop oncoming traffic. (If you're stretching your right side, lock with the left arm; and vice versa.) Stop when the arm is perpendicular to your body. Ideally, fingers should be uncurled, reaching toward the ceiling and back toward the body. Hold it there with the fingers arched back. That's a strong "stop" sign. You should feel the wrist stretch while you're sweeping your hand out to the side; it continues to hurt while the coach applies weight. Always return your arm to the starting postition at your side before beginning the next repetition. Make sure that you maintain a good stop sign throughout a workout. Work as hard the last time you do a stop sign as you did the first time.

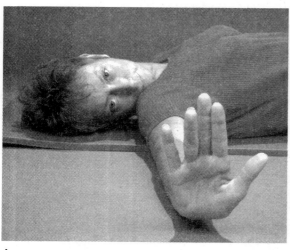
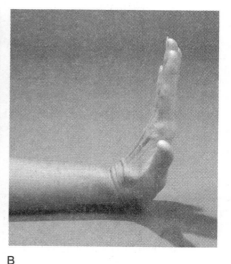

A   B

Figure 8.1   Stop Sign

2. At the same time, pull the toes of both feet back toward your head and push your heels away from your butt as far as you can. Hold them there. Keep your heels resting on the floor. Relax your back. (The feet are bare in figure 8.2 to show how much of a reach should be taking place.)

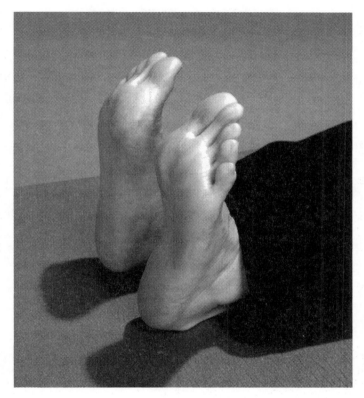

Figure 8.2   Foot Lock

3. As your arm is fully extending and heels are pointing out, slowly roll your head toward your outstretched arm and point your nose down toward your shoulder. When you begin, your head should be resting in a neutral position with the nose toward the ceiling (figure 8.3A). Do not lift the head off the floor. Just roll it slowly and smoothly toward your shoulder (figure 8.3B). Make sure you tuck your nose down to your shoulder while you keep your eyes open. You should feel a distinct pull on the opposite side of your neck. Hold it there (figure 8.3C). If you don't feel this pull, your nose isn't far enough over toward your shoulder. Don't pick up the head and reposition it; doing

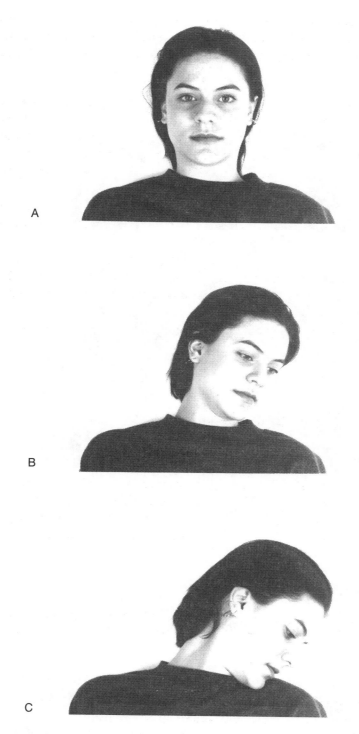

Figure 8.3   Head Roll

so may put a crink in your neck. You get a more powerful stretch if you roll your head after your coach applies weight. Hold it there. (Some people, but only a few, need a pillow to support the back of the head.)

If your back hurts, it's usually because you're trying too hard or are arching your back. Do not arch your back. Keep your heels on the floor. You should feel most of the Lock in the back of your legs, not your back.

You are now Locked—toes pointing inward toward your body, arm at a 90-degree angle from your body, palm facing out like a stop sign, and head and nose pointed down toward your shoulder.

You will hold this Lock throughout each stretch. Your Coach will tell you if you're slacking off—how and where. Go back and find the Lock, because the payoff will be a more effective stretch.

At the end of each stretch, Un-Lock by returning to a relaxed position with feet loose, arms at your sides, and nose pointed up. **Do not lift up the head to Un-Lock**. Roll it back to a straight position, and slide your arm along the floor back to your side.

When you're ready, Lock again for the next stretch. Remember: A good Lock is the key to a good stretch.

Important Tips for the PIC

Keep these tips in mind every time you stretch.

- ▶ The amount of pain relief you'll get depends entirely on how hard you work on these stretches. Don't be a wimp. Really *feel* each stretch and go after whatever pain is inside your body. Only by stretching out the connective tissue will you shoo pain out of your body.

- ▶ Do all of the stretches *slowly*.

- ▶ Keep your eyes open so your coach can assess how you're doing. This will be hard to do, because your natural inclination is to close your eyes and grit your teeth. Don't do it! Stay alert! Stay awake! Stay aware!

- ▶ Remember to keep breathing. Just breathe normally. When you breathe normally, the coach can see when you're working hard and when you're not. If you're breathing too easily, it means you're not working hard enough. The coach should notice a slight sense of struggle as a sign that you're breathing normally but hard enough to make the stretch work.

➤ No gum-chewing is allowed during a workout. Chewing gum while on your back is a perfect opportunity to choke.

➤ Know that you'll get the best results if all drugs—over-the-counter painkillers, alcohol, prescription drugs—are out of your body. Even caffeine can dull your senses, and too much of it will affect how well you'll be able to feel the stretches inside your tissue. So try to be drug-free and caffeine-free when you stretch. Okay, I admit it. I'm a coffee-crazed latte bug. You can take the coffee warning lightly, but if you drink lots of coffee and can't feel a difference after doing the stretches, cutting back or eliminating caffeine can make a huge impact.

➤ Before you begin a workout, compare one side of your body to the other. Roll your arms and wrists. Bend your elbows at the same time toward your body. Do it lying down or standing. To determine how and where these stretches work, you need a starting point for how your body feels—where it's loose, where it's tight, where it hurts the most. Then when you stretch, start first on your "good" side—the one that hurts least. Trust me on this one. Starting on the good side gives you something against which to compare the other side of your body. Frequent comparisons will help you feel how the stretches are loosening your body and easing your pain. The pain may be most bothersome on your bad side, but working the good side first gives you impetus and encouragement to go after the painful side with even more gusto because you'll know what to expect. And gusto is good!

➤ If possible take a walk for about five minutes after your workout. While you walk, continue your comparisons. Roll your wrists, bend your elbows, feel how you hold your shoulders. Search for areas of looseness and tightness throughout your upper body. Ideally, your arms should hang loosely from your shoulders, as if they're dangling like a marionette's arms. When you stop walking, your arms should feel limp and relaxed. That feeling of looseness is your goal.

➤

Important Tips for the Coach

Keep these tips in mind every time you stretch.

➤ Really, truly play the role of a coach. Encourage your partner. Make your partner work at these stretches. Growl if you must. Keep up a constant chatter of instructions and challenges. Here are some examples:

Work it out. Come on! Stretch it!

Keep those fingers reaching! Stre-eeeetch!

Go for it! Lock! Do it, do it, do it!

Keep your eyes open! Breathe!

Slowly, slowly. Reach for the door. No cheating!

➤ Be imaginative, supportive, and coach-like.

➤ Use a chair for balance. There's no need for *you* to develop aches or pains by helping someone else get rid of his or hers. There's no need for you to fall on your best buddy during a workout (and squashed friends make terrible references). Remember, use the chair for balance only. Do not lean on it. Do not depend on it. Make sure it's the proper height, meaning you don't have to reach up or down to grasp the back of it. If the chair is too high or too low, your back will begin to hurt. Stand up straight. Tilt your head down to look at the person; don't bend from the waist. Doing so will give you a backache very quickly.

➤ If you find yourself in the wrong position during a workout or while you're applying weight with your foot, *do not hop* to another position. I repeat; do not hop. Stop what you're doing, remove your foot from the PIC's body, stand on both feet and then reposition yourself. You wouldn't want someone to hop while his or her foot is firmly planted on you, would you?

➤ Always make sure your partner Locks before doing the stretch. Locking is one of the keys to the effectiveness of these workouts. (Hint: Your partner may try to cheat by loosening up or not Locking completely. Be alert! PICs often cheat after the first stretch that uncovers a lot of pain; they'll try to slack off on the very next stretch.) Constantly remind your partner during the stretch to stay Locked—toes pointed toward the body, arm out straight like a stop sign, and head rolled to the side with nose pointed toward the shoulder.

➤ Be aware of your stance. You body should be relaxed and erect. Hold the back of a chair for balance. Keep the arm nearest the PIC's head free to demonstrate movements or stretches to your partner. You should be able to see your PIC from head to toe and complete all the cross-checks needed during each stretch. Make sure you're standing up straight. Tilt your head down to look at the PIC. Don't lean. Don't bend from the waist. If you do these techniques while you're bent over, you'll get a neckache or backache. Be vertical, relax your shoulders, and you'll be fine. Remember: You should feel relaxed while helping with the workout.

▸ Don't turn your head downward excessively during the stretches. (What's excessive? If you have a backache the next day, you were tilting or leaning excessively.)

▸ Time each stretch for ten seconds from the moment the Lock is in place. If the PIC feels the need for a little more stretching, allow it.

▸ Use the same foot on the same side of your partner's body (right foot to apply weight on the PIC's right arm or shoulder, left foot on the PIC's left arm or shoulder).

▸ Your *Working* foot applies weight. Your *Base* foot stabilizes you as you add weight.

▸ Apply the weight straight down, not from an angle, with your Working foot. Extend the toes upward on your Working foot when applying weight. It takes less effort to add weight and help with the stretch if your toes are arched.

▸ Encourage the PIC to take a walk after each workout.

▸ When each stretch is finished, use your toes and the ball of your foot to make a few small, slow, light twists on the skin where you just finished a technique to reduce the residual tingling left over from the stretch or stretches. Do this for about thirty seconds. This is called applying a Tiny Torque. Or use your hands to apply Mr. Twister. See Chapter 10 for full instructions on applying Tiny Torque or Mr. Twister.

How These Stretches Got Their Names

Why do these stretches have names like Mr. Twister and Windshield Wiper? When I first began using these stretches with clients, I didn't keep track of names because I was interested only in results. But when I started teaching them to others, questions inevitably arose. What's this called? Why do you do it this way and not that way? What's it called when you do this a different way?

Soon, it was clear that every technique and variation had to have a name, especially when I was consulting with people by phone. It became increasingly difficult to describe the techniques, particularly if people had not seen them before or were inexperienced at using them. By naming the techniques, everyone had a base of knowledge and a platform of definitions.

Once the techniques had names, other people knew what I was talking about and what they were supposed to do. The names became descriptive of what each technique involved. Because my audience is the general public, I chose simple, descriptive names. Thanks to all who suggested and contributed ideas!

Chapter 9

How to Know If You're Doing These Stretches Correctly

Since these stretches are new and somewhat unusual-looking to you, you'll probably have questions about whether you're doing them right. How will you know if you're doing a particular stretch properly? How will your coach know?

Cross-checking:
The Coach's Job

Cross-checking is a term that describes frequent, quick assessments by the coach to monitor and assess the effectiveness of each technique in progress. Basically, the coach periodically does a triangular, visual sweep of the PIC's body—checks the feet, head, and arms—to make sure everything's being done correctly for an optimum stretch. Here's what you should pay attention to:

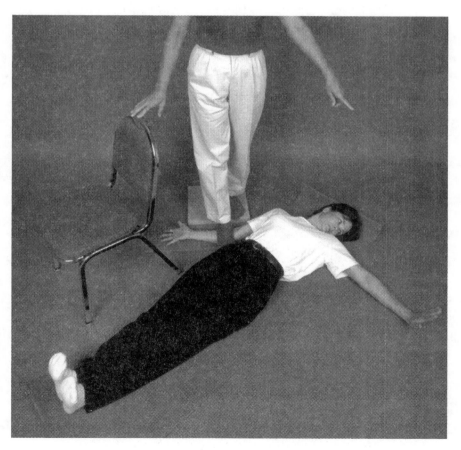

Figure 9.1   Cross-check

Feet. The PIC's feet should be Locked, with toes pointing toward the head and heels pushed out away from the butt. No slacking off allowed. Keep reminding the PIC to Lock the feet.

Reminder: The Locking movement involves the feet only, not the back. The PIC's back should not look as if it's been tightened. If it does look that way, ask the PIC to un-Lock and start over, keeping the back relaxed. Focus only on the feet.

Hand/arm position during the Lock. The PIC's Locked arm should be perpendicular to the body, hand out as if it's stopping oncoming traffic (see figure 8.1), fingers straight and pointing toward the ceiling. Don't let the hand tilt or roll to the side, or the fingers curl. (During the back stretches, make sure the hands stay flat on the stomach, palms down, and watch for squeezing, curled fingers, or tight-fisted grips as evidence of how hard the PIC is working.)

Nose-shoulder-head. The PIC's head should be turned toward the Locked arm/shoulder with the nose pointed down toward the shoulder. Keep reminding the PIC to turn the nose down to the shoulder. Make sure this is done by rolling the head, not by lifting it and placing it to the side. Done properly, the nose will roll over to the shoulder automatically and then tilt down a little farther. That's the desired position (see figure 8.3).

Eyes. When people think about or experience pain, they often close their eyes or wince really hard. It's important during the Rossiter System stretches for the PIC to keep his or her eyes open. That way, you can interpret what's going on inside the PIC's body and how much pain the PIC is feeling. You must be aware of the PIC's movements and progress during each stretch. The eyes tell whether the PIC is working or not.

Breathing. You need to remind the PIC to breathe, as many people in pain often hold their breath. Watch the PIC's stomach for up-and-down movement that shows the lungs are working. If the stomach is flat and steady, issue constant reminders to breathe. Remember, the body and its tissues need a constant supply of oxygen! When PICs hold their breath, they're holding you out, which means the stretching work isn't getting done.

Verbal feedback/comparisons. Ask for feedback in ways that force the PIC to identify and specify whether he or she feels "better" or "worse" after a certain technique or series of stretches. Know this: Your time will be wasted if all your PIC says after a stretch is, "It feels different." In my estimation, "different" is a vague answer, so don't accept it. "Different" gives the PIC no incentive to keep stretching. "Different" means the PIC might not be willing to work hard at these techniques or accept responsibility for positive change.

If your PIC offers vague answers, ask open-ended but pointed questions to help the PIC focus on the specific bodily changes that are (or are not) occurring. Don't put words in the PIC's mouth. Ask questions that are helpful. (For example: "How does it feel different?" "Does it feel lighter or heavier?" "Does it move more freely or less freely?" "Is the sting less or more intensive?" "Has the numbness shifted or disappeared?" "What does it feel like now compared with ten minutes ago?" "How does this arm feel compared to the arm that hasn't been stretched yet?")

Remember: This is a team effort. Coaches need to know how their players (PICs) are faring and feeling in order to keep coaching well.

I can't stress enough the importance of comparing. For me, comparing is an everyday thing. I compare grocery stores. Does the store have what I want? How long do I have to wait in line? Most stores stock the same products, so I choose the one with the shortest checkout lines.

What I'm asking you to do with these stretches is a simple before-and-after comparison of your body. You own it, and your body's loaded with information. Compare your right side to your left side. Compare the front of your body to the back, your right arm to your left arm. Is one lighter or heavier? Which one moves better? Do they hurt in different places? Do they hurt at the same time? When do they hurt? Stop what you're doing right now and *feel*. If you had to pick one side over the other, which side would you pick. Why?

Make these comparisons a part of your continuing workouts. The woman in figure 9.1 is comparing her elbows.

Tissue. This crosscheck is called *Tissue Wisdom*. Remember, from chapter 2, how it's possible to feel in someone's nose the movement of connective tissue in his or her fingers or toes? As you do these stretches, you will become better at feeling when connective tissue has moved and stretched to its fullest potential.

Connective tissue and underlying muscles are amazing in that they can tell you when they are "done" stretching. As a coach, you will know the precise feeling under your PIC's skin.

When you first begin the stretches, you will feel under your foot the back-and-forth movement of the PIC's tissue and muscles. That's an indication that the PIC is stretching. When doing the first technique, Forearm Up, for example, the PIC moves and waves the fingers slowly. What you will feel under your foot is the PIC's forearm tissue sliding and moving toward and then away from the elbow with each wiggle and wave. Eventually, the back-and-forth movement will change to an up-and-down movement, and when you get that signal, the tissue is "home" and no longer needs help. The area is "done."

It may sound strange now, but in time, you'll get the feel of Tissue Wisdom. Just remember to feel and pay attention to how your PIC's body moves, responds, relaxes, and stretches. In time, you'll be a pro—and so will your foot. Don't forget that the sensation of being "home" exists only underneath the place your foot last worked. Other areas nearby or deeper still may need to be stretched and worked out, so it's important to be comprehensive. Feet rule, Coaches. Listen to your feet.

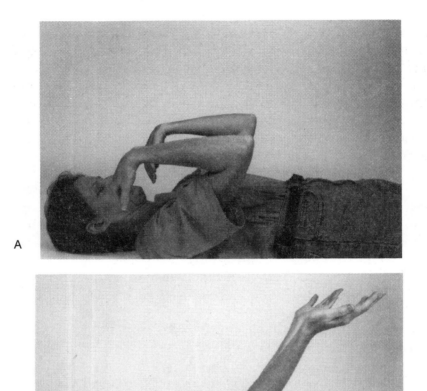

Figure 9.2   Elbow Comparison

Paying Attention: The PIC's Job

As the PIC, it's important to pay attention to how your body feels before each stretch so there's a standard for comparison afterward. Pay attention to tightness, ease or difficulty of movement, heaviness or lightness, tingling or numbness in your hands, fingers, arms, shoulders, head, and neck. Really grasp how your body feels so you'll know what you're working toward at the end of a stretch. If a wrist feels sore or tight, for example, understand that you're stretching it to feel pain-free and fluid after a stretch.

Always begin on the "good" side. Here's another reason to pay attention to how your body feels before and after the stretches. I always encourage people to begin stretching first on the side of their body that hurts less than the other. If you begin stretching your "good" side first, you'll get accustomed to the feel, discomfort level, and the amount of work needed to make these workouts produce positive results. That way, when you move to the hurting, or "bad," side of your body, you'll know what to expect—and how much effort will be involved. If pain is too intense, you'll know when to ease up or stop.

Listen to your body. It is a powerful communicator.

Chapter 10

The Rossiter Stretches for the Upper Body

You'll Feel Good: The Effects of Rossiter Stretches

In a few minutes, you'll begin the Rossiter stretches. After completing the first few, pay attention to your body and how it feels. Many people feel looser, lighter, freer, and less achy as soon as they complete these stretches. Others may notice slight differences. Some may not notice anything at all, not the first time anyway. Typically, people who feel no difference after stretching have been using nonsteroidal anti-inflammatory drugs (NSAIDs), have had shots, or have undergone surgery. Or the pain is so overwhelming, they haven't made a dent yet.

These stretches can be done several times a week for the first few weeks until all the residual pain is worked out of your body and the connective tissue is restored to its natural state. Once you've reached that point, using the stretches becomes a matter of maintenance, something to do every week or so, once a month, or whenever aches and pains signal their return.

Some people will notice bruises a day or two after doing a Rossiter workout. Tissue usually bruises for any (or all) of the following reasons:

Speed. If you wiggled your fingers too fast or hurried through the techniques, it's quite possible you'll bruise. Closely follow the directions for each technique and do each of the stretching sets *slowly* and *deliberately*. Once you're proficient at the stretches, you and your coach should be able to do all the upper-body stretches correctly and slowly in 20–30 minutes.

Too Much Weight Too Quickly. Some people will bruise no matter how much weight is added. It's up to the coach to add weight slowly and safely. That's why communication between coach and PIC is so important—the PIC needs to let the coach know how much weight is enough, and the coach needs to develop a feel for how much the PIC can handle. Talk to each other. Watch each other's body language. Re-read chapter 4 for tips and guidelines on weight.

The Number of Techniques Performed. Connective tissue responds best when the techniques are done three times each with the right amount of weight (that means as much as the PIC can take). If the PIC can handle more weight but chooses not to, chances are the technique will have to be done more than the recommended three times to get the same results, and doing a specific stretch six or eight times, for example, will cause bruises. It's a simple matter of overuse.

What if you do fewer than three stretches? Recovery from your pain will take longer. If you're working with someone older (meaning chronologically old, fragile, or both), sets of two may be fine. If you're working with people in their sixties, seventies, or eighties and don't know them personally, it might be wise to take it easy and start with two repetitions instead of three.

If you want to do each stretch four times, make sure you know your capability. Doing four can produce soreness for a while, but for many people, soreness is better than pain. And if soreness develops, you can always use Tiny Torques and Mr. Twisters (which you'll read about soon) to relieve it.

The best advice is to work up to a level of capability slowly, especially until you get a feel for what these stretches can do. No need to be macho or overly brave about your pain. Three stretches are thorough, and three stretches are enough. Do the techniques slowly, properly, with enough weight and three times each on both sides, and you should do just fine.

Reminders Before You Begin

Keep the following tips in mind when you're stretching.

- ➤ Keep breathing as you stretch.

- ➤ Keep your eyes open. It's the best way to make sure coach and PIC are communicating and paying attention to each other's body signals.

- ➤ Do these stretches slowly. Do not hurry or speed through them. Your pain has built up slowly, and you need to stretch it away slowly.

- ➤ Consciously stretch away your pain. Don't be wimpy!

- ➤ Maintain the Lock throughout the stretch.

- ➤ Do these as a series of stretches, not as individual spot stretches. They are meant to stretch out your body's system of connective tissue, not isolated bits and pieces.

- ➤ During and between stretches, occasionally shake out and bend your arms, wrists, hands, and shoulders to compare your body's stretched side with the unstretched side.

- ➤ The coach applies weight, not pressure, with the foot. Flex the toes upward when adding weight.

- ➤ The PIC accepts as much weight as possible. Talk frequently if weight needs to be added or lessened.

- ➤ Do each technique three times. With each stretch, the coach moves the foot 1/4-inch in the direction specified.

- ➤ Do all five floor stretches (Forearm Up, Forearm Down, Bicep, Bicep Torque, and Hole in the Shoulder) on both sides of the PIC's body. After both sides have been stretched, move to a straight-back chair for the final stretch, Traps.

Tiny Torque and Mr. Twister, the Soothing Components of the Rossiter System

It's quite possible that the Rossiter stretches will cause momentary tingling or soreness in the PIC's muscles. A workout can also produce lingering or residual pain, even the day after they've been done. When that happens, it's time to apply a Tiny Torque or use Mr. Twister!

Tiny Torque

Tiny Torque means just that—a tiny torquing or turning motion on a just-stretched muscle that hurts. It provides relief by soothing and warming the tissue until it quits twitching, buzzing, or stinging. Some people need a soothing Tiny Torque after each stretch; others need it as they learn the stretches, but the need tapers off as they become more proficient at stretching.

Here's how Tiny Torque works:

What the PIC Does

1. As soon as the coach removes the foot after a technique, you will be able to tell if there is lingering pain or stinging. If there is, the coach can do a Tiny Torque, by very gently re-applying the foot to your muscle using the area of the foot from the ball to the toes.

2. Tell your coach when the stinging has subsided. It may take thirty seconds or more until your muscles feel soothed. You may even need to ask your coach to repeat the Tiny Torque.

What the Coach Does

1. Start with your heel turned out or in (as in figure 10.1A) and place the ball of your foot on the sore tissue.

2. Press lightly and turn the heel back to a normal position (as in figure 10.1B) with a downward turning or rotating motion. The PIC's skin should turn with your foot. Do it gently! Use about one pound of pressure—that means a very *light* touch. Figure 10.1 shows the Tiny Torque being done on the forearm.

Hint: This is not a rub. You are lightly turning the tissue using the ball of your foot and then holding it in place. The torque should literally suck the pain or sting out of the PIC's tissue.

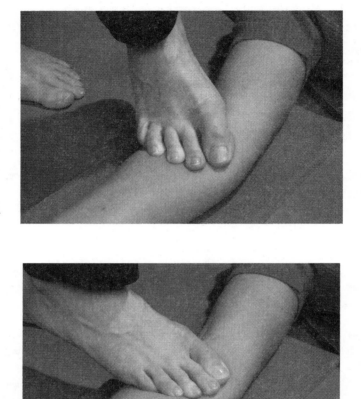

A

B

Figure 10.1   Tiny Torque

3. Continue to apply the Tiny Torque for at least thirty seconds. Your PIC will tell you when the sting is gone. If the sting doesn't disappear after thirty seconds, repeat the Tiny Torque. Move your foot to cover the entire area. However, if the PIC is still hurting after a full stretching session in which you've consistently delivered Tiny Torques, tell the PIC to lie on the ground and then go to work. Tiny Torque all over again, wherever it hurts.

4. As you apply a Tiny Torque, you may feel a light twinge or pulsing in the tissue that's just been stretched. With each Tiny Torque, you may actually feel the PIC's tissue relaxing. It's almost as if you can feel the underlying tissue go "aaaaahhhh" as it finds its way back home. Be aware of this sensation. Get accustomed to how it feels.

Mr. Twister

Mr. Twister provides the same kind of relief as a Tiny Torque but with two differences: Mr. Twister is applied with the hands, and it provides relief over a greater area of tissue and muscle than a Tiny Torque. Use Mr. Twister to soothe any area that's still smarting or stinging after you've completed all the floor stretches. It's not a specific stretch like the other techniques, but it sucks out lingering soreness from and calms an area that's already been stretched. It can be done in a standing or seated position.

Here's how it works:

What the PIC Does

1. Sitting in a chair, identify the area that still hurts, stings, or is sore. For this example, let's say it's an arm.

2. Try to relax completely.

3. As your coach does Mr. Twister on you, pay attention to how your tissue feels. Tell your coach when the stinging or soreness subsides.

What the Coach Does

1. Use both hands and take the PIC's arm where the pain is. Hold it as though you are about to wring out a towel. Your hands should be only two to four inches apart, with one covering the top of the PIC's arm and the other covering the bottom (as in figure 10.2A).

2. With each hand, turn the tissue in different directions very lightly toward the center (as in figure 10.2B).

3. Hold the twist for about 30 seconds.

4. Move your hands slightly up from the area you've just Mr. Twister-ed and repeat. Hold each area until the PIC feels a difference in the tissue and the stinging/soreness subsides.

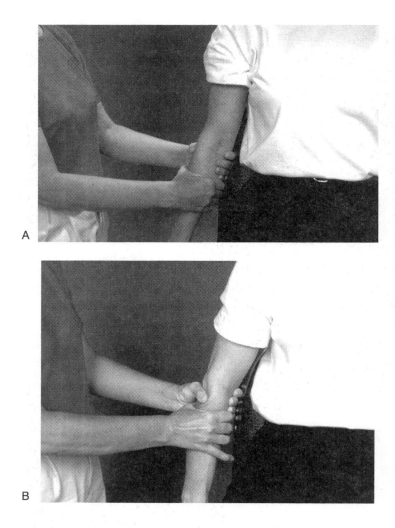

Figure 10.2   Mr. Twister

Hint: The PIC's body must not be tense. The arm or area being worked on must be relaxed or this is an exercise in futility. Do not let the PIC "help" you by holding up or tensing the area being worked on (as in figure 10.3). Any muscle tension in the area wastes your time. Make sure the PIC's arms are floppy at the side.

---

5. As you apply the twist, you may notice that the underlying tissue relaxes. The more experienced you get, the sooner you'll feel the underlying tissue go "aaaaahhhhh." It means you've done well.

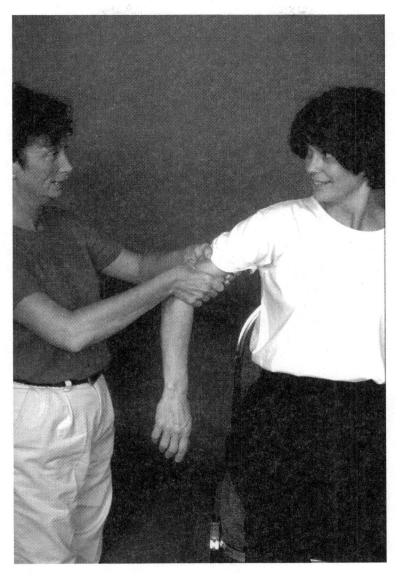

Figure 10.3   The Wrong Way to Do Mr. Twister

Mr. Twister isn't used as often as Tiny Torque. The more the PIC becomes used to the feel of a workout, the less she needs Tiny Torque or Mr. Twister.

You're now ready to start the Rossiter System series of stretches.

Note: Throughout these stretches, pronouns will take turns between "him" and "her" to avoid awkward sentences.

Stretch 1: Forearm Up

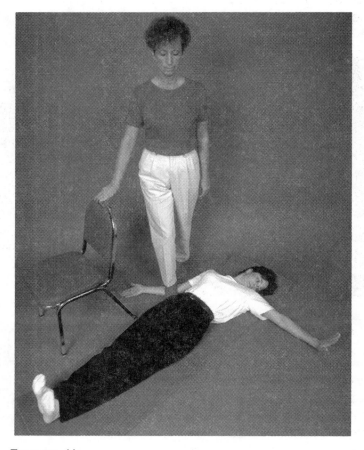

Figure 10.4   Forearm Up

What the PIC Does

1. Lie face up on a protective mat. Relax. Take a deep breath.

2. Place your arm at a 45-degree angle from your body, as in figure 10.5A. (Imagine your feet as the 6 on a clock face and your head as the 12, pointing your arm between the 4 and 5 or 7 and 8, depending on which arm you're stretching. That's about 45 degrees.)

3. Make sure the palm of your hand is exactly face up and flat on the mat, as in figure 10.5B, so that the two bones of your forearm are parallel to the floor and mat. If the thumb is too high, the bones will not rest properly on the floor.

Hint: If this position strains the elbow or shoulder, move the hand farther away from the body to make sure the forearm bones are parallel to the floor.

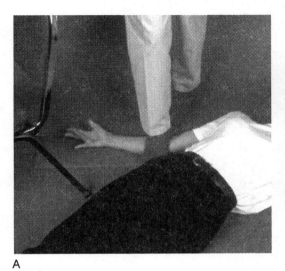

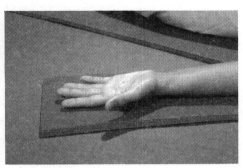

A

B

Figure 10.5   Forearm Close-up

4. Your coach will apply weight slowly with his or her foot to your forearm just below the elbow. Let the Coach know when it's enough weight by saying "Stop!" or "Enough!" How will you know it's enough? It'll feel uncomfortable. Just make sure the Coach gives you enough weight and it remains steady. Don't make your muscle hard to stop the coach from adding weight or to avoid discomfort. Doing so stops the process cold. Relax the arm!

Hint: How does "uncomfortable" feel? It means more than the first sign of pain, more than a little tenderness. It's enough weight to open your eyes wide. It's enough weight to make you think, "If she puts just one more ounce on me, I'll yank this arm!" You should think about whining when it's enough. It's a fine whine, so let it age. Reread the section in chapter 4 for a refresher on weight.

5. When the coach tells you to Lock, tilt your toes up toward your nose as if pushing your heels away from your butt and slide your other arm up along the floor out to shoulder height. Your palm should be facing out, as if making a gesture to stop oncoming traffic, fingers

pointed toward the ceiling. At the same time, gently roll your head away from your coach and point your nose down toward your shoulder. You can review the Locking instructions in chapter 8 if you need to. Remember to roll your head; don't lift it. Lifting it will unnecessarily strain the neck. Maintain this Lock throughout the stretch. If you feel yourself slacking off—if your toes quit reaching, your arm wimps out, or your head begins to loosen and turn upward—go back and find the Lock. Stay Locked during the entire stretch!

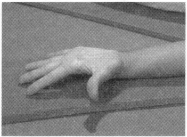

A   Hard Stretch

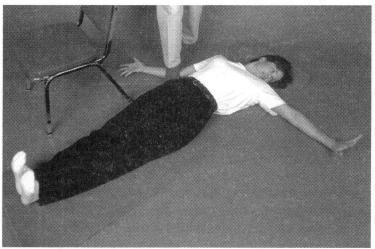

B   Hard Stretch with Full Lock

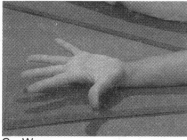

C   Wave

Figure 10.6   Forearm Up

6. Keep your eyes open! Breathe!

7. When your coach tells you to begin stretching, spread out the fingers of the arm being stepped on, as in figure 10.6A and B. Slowly move those fingers like a rolling wave, one finger at a time, with the hand outstretched as far out as you can, as in figure 10.6C. Wave *slowly*. Move each finger independently, all the while reaching outward, stretching, flexing, and rippling it slowly, deliberately. Make sure to include the thumb. If you find a certain spot or finger that's tender or more sensitive than others, stay with that spot for a moment and really reach and stretch. Remember, you have to *feel* this to make it work! Stretch for 10 seconds, which your coach will count. When the stretch is over, your coach will remove her foot from your arm.

Hint: If you Lock properly, the act of Locking will make the area under the foot feel like more weight has been added. If you stretch out your fingers properly, the area under your coach's foot should again feel like weight has been added to your arm.

---

8. When your coach removes her foot from your forearm, take a breath and relax the arm. Un-Lock by returning your outstretched arm to your side and relaxing your head and shoulder. Your other arm stays at a 45° angle on the mat. If you need to rest, tell the coach.

When you're ready to begin again, your coach will place her foot 1/4-inch down your arm and add weight again for another stretch. It'll be easier this time because you're overlapping the stretch on another part of the arm. However, if the next stretches are more painful than the first, it means there's more pain embedded in the muscle and connective tissue than you thought. You will do a total of three stretches, each time taking an appropriate amount of weight to help you find the pain and stretch it out. Listen to your body. Work through the tender and painful areas by stretching as much as you can.

What the Coach Does

1. The foot that applies weight is your Working foot. The other foot, the Back, or Base, foot, stays behind you for balance and steadiness. Place the arch of your Working foot 1/2-inch below the PIC's elbow. (Remember: Same side, same foot. If it's your partner's right arm, use your right foot. Left arm, use your left foot.) Apply weight by lifting off the Base foot and rolling forward onto the Working foot. Roll up and onto the ball of your Base foot to give the proper amount of

weight to the PIC's arm. The straighter your working knee, the better. If your PIC is large or has bulky arms or shoulders, you might want to use a stand to add weight more effectively. This stand allows both of your feet to stay at the same level while adding weight. The stand allows you to roll your Working foot onto the PIC's arm while keeping your knee straight. Simply rock off your Base foot and add weight with your Working foot.

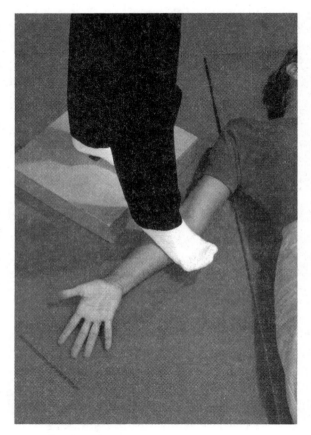

Figure 10.7   Forearm Up with Stand

Hint: Place a chair next to you for balance. Do not lean on it. Do not hop when changing position. Simply use it to steady yourself.

---

2. Curl up the toes of your Working foot, as in figure 10.8, and apply weight straight down onto the PIC's arm approximately 1/2-inch below the elbow joint. Never step on a joint. The exact spot you choose is your call. Add weight slowly and smoothly until the PIC

tells you it's enough with "Stop!" or "Enough!" When the PIC winces, you'll know it's enough weight.

Hint: Apply weight slowly enough so the PIC isn't inclined to yank his arm out and away. The PIC must *tell* you when to stop; making grimacing faces isn't good enough.

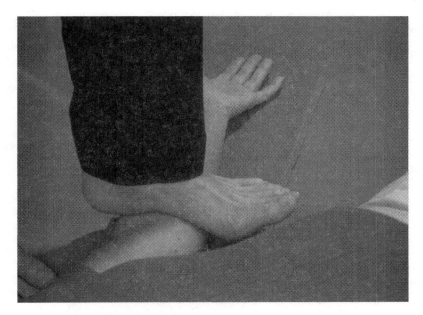

Figure 10.8   Toes Up, Weight Down

3. As soon as the weight is applied, ask the PIC to Lock by flexing his toes toward his nose and pushing the heels away from the butt. At the same time, the PIC will slide the opposite arm straight out to the side along the floor to shoulder height with the palm facing out, like a stop sign. The PIC's fingers should point toward the ceiling. Ask him to roll his head toward the shoulder of the outstretched arm and hold the Lock there. With your free hand, point to the critical Locking areas—the toes, the arm, the shoulder, and head—to remind your PIC to stay Locked.

4. Begin counting to 10 after you apply the weight.

5. Ask your PIC to begin stretching by slowly and individually waving the fingers of the hand to which you're applying weight, reaching outward with each finger. Make sure it's a slow, deliberate, rippling

wave with finger reaches that are good and strong (see figure 10.6). In the bottom of your foot you should be able to feel movement from your partner's hand stretches. A wimpy reach will not produce ripples that you can feel. A good, effective reach will create definite powerful movement in the connective tissue and muscles of the PIC's forearm. If your PIC is really working, the skin on his palm will turn whitish from the tissue being stretched underneath. That's good! Encourage more of it! If you feel the PIC slack off, use cheers and words of encouragement to keep the stretch going. Keep talking, keep reminding.

6. Cross-check: Make sure the Lock stays in place throughout the stretch. Remind the PIC to point toes, breathe, keep the Locking arm out straight, turn the head toward the shoulder, as in figure 10.9, point the nose downward, and stretch. Cheer him on. Keep talking. Make sure you keep breathing, too.

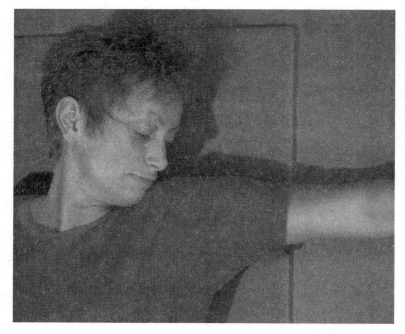

Figure 10.9   Forearm Up Head Roll in Locked Position

7. After you've counted 10 seconds, tell the PIC to relax and then remove your foot from his forearm.

8. Take a breath and encourage your PIC to do the same.

9. Good job! You've completed your first Rossiter Technique!

To complete a Forearm Up set, do this stretch a total of three times. Each time, move your foot 1/4-inch farther down the PIC's arm (toward the wrist but always in the fleshy, muscle part of the upper third of the forearm).

Stretch 2: Forearm Down

Forearm Down is similar to Forearm Up, but this part of your forearm usually doesn't need as much work (not always, anyway). This spot may be more tender than the area worked in Forearm Up, so be aware that the PIC may not take as much weight.

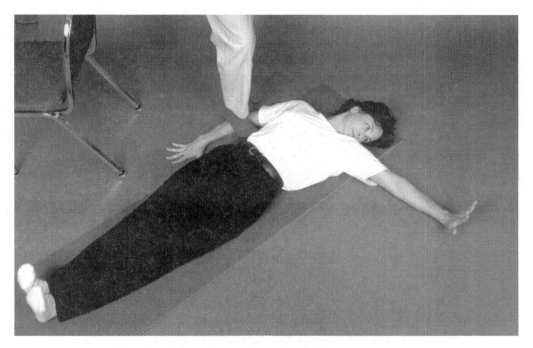

Figure 10.10   Forearm Down

What the PIC Does

1. Lie face up on the mat. Take a deep breath and relax.

2. Place your arm, palm down, parallel to your body with a slight but noticeable bend in your elbow. This allows the two bones of the lower arm to lie parallel instead of crossing each other.

3. Allow your coach to apply weight slowly, just below your elbow (the same spot as in Forearm Up). Take as much weight as you can.

4. When the weight is applied, Lock and maintain the Lock when the Coach tells you to (as in figure 10.10).

5. As soon as the Lock is in place, spread out the fingers of the hand being stretched. Move them like a wave, slowly, deliberately, individually. Feel the stretch in each finger, the palm, and lower your forearm. If you find a tender or sensitive spot, go after it! Feel the stretch and take it as far as it will go. Keep the stretched-out palm parallel to the floor. Keep stretching and waving while your coach counts to 10.

6. When the coach removes her foot from your forearm, breathe and relax the arm. Shake it out if you feel the need. Return your Locked arm to your side, relax your head and shoulder, and return your nose skyward. Both shoulders should be down and relaxed.

What the Coach Does

1. Make sure the PIC's palm is facing down and arm is parallel to the rest of his body, with the elbow bent noticeably.

2. Encourage the PIC to take a deep breath and relax the arm.

3. Curl up the toes of your Working foot and apply weight straight down onto your PIC's forearm, one inch below the elbow, as in figure 10.11. Do not add weight on any joints! Stay in the fleshy part of the arm. Use the arch of your foot, close to the heel. Apply the weight slowly. Keep asking, "Can you handle a little more weight?" When your PIC lets you know, stop adding weight.

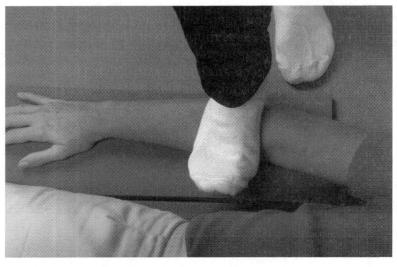

Figure 10.11   Forearm Down (Close-up)

Hint: Use a stand whenever possible (as in figure 10.12); it makes it easier to balance especially if the PIC is large-muscled, large-boned, or just plain bigger than the coach.

---

4. Tell your PIC to Lock. When the Lock is in place, begin counting to 10.

5. Ask your PIC to slowly, gently, and deliberately begin stretching the hand of the arm on which you're standing. Make sure the reach can be felt in the bottom of your foot; if you feel nothing, your PIC isn't working hard enough. Egg him on! Look for winces and whitish tissue on the hand, palm, and fingers as signs of a good stretch.

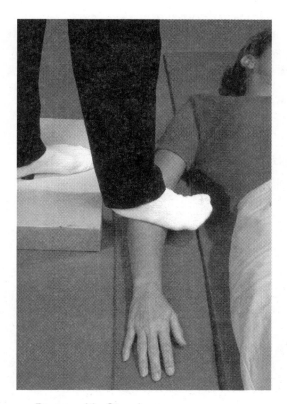

Figure 10.12   Forearm Down with Stand

6. Cross-check: Make sure the Lock stays in place. Encourage! Coach!

7. When you've reached a ten count, tell the PIC to relax and remove your foot from the forearm. Make sure the PIC returns the Locked arm to the side and relaxes the head and shoulder.

8. Take a breath and encourage your PIC to do the same.

Repeat the stretch two more times. Each time, moves your foot 1/4-inch down the PIC's arm.

Hint: After a really good Forearm Down stretch, a Tiny Torque can be quite refreshing. As coach, you'll win friends and influence people by doing one or two torques automatically.

Stretch 3: The Bicep

The next four techniques provide more long-term relief than the first two. Now that you're more sensitive to pain in the tissue, you'll be able to recognize the type of pain you're trying to get out of your body and the type of pain you're trying to avoid.

While this stretch is a bit more painful, it's also a lot more fruitful. Work hard at it. You'll be amazed at the results.

What The PIC Does

1. Lie face up on the mat. Take a deep breath and relax.

2. Place your arm at a 30-degree angle from the body so that your palm is facing exactly up. If this hurts your elbow or shoulder, move the hand farther away from your body to make sure the forearm bones are parallel to the floor.

3. The coach will gently place his foot on your biceps, about 1 inch above your elbow. When the foot is in place, bring your hand straight up and gently place it against the calf of your coach's leg—fingers straight up, palm flat (as in figure 10.13A). Don't curve your hand around your coach's leg, and make sure that your thumb is away from the leg.

4. The coach slowly will add weight to your biceps. This area may be tender, but take *almost* as much weight as you can. *Don't take a maximum amount of weight, because this is a hard stretch.* You'll find out why very soon.

5. When the coach tells you, Lock up and maintain the Lock throughout the stretch.

6. When the 10-count begins, *very* slowly peel your hand back and away from the coach's calf, leading with the tips of your fingers (as in figure

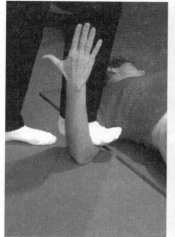

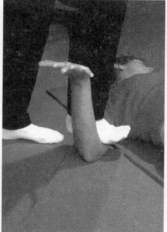

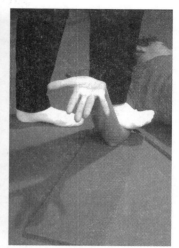

A   Bicep Start   B   Fingers Arch Back   C   Wrist Leaves Leg

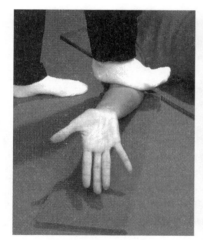

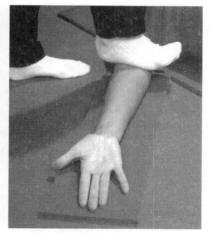

D   Fingers Touch Floor   E Flattened Wrist

Figure 10.13   The Bicep

10.13B). As soon as the palm is arched back as far as it can go, slowly straighten your elbow, reaching back with your fingertips (as in figure 10.3C). Return the hand to where it was on the floor before the stretch. Keep the arm pulled in toward your body, not out and away. *Very* slowly, keep peeling the hand back toward the floor, as if you're peeling a banana. This is *hard* work. Remember to lead with your fingertips. Your goal is to lay the back of your hand and arm flat on the floor. When your fingertips reach the carpet or pad (as in figure 10.13D), bring the wrist down to the floor to join your fingers (as in figure 10.13E). Maintain the stretch until the wrist flattens to the floor (not the fingers or the knuckles—the *wrist*). This last little bit is tough! Go after it! Consciously *stretch* out the soreness and pain.

Hint: Keep in mind that this is a distance technique. It should take about 10 seconds for your arm to cover the distance from the coach's calf to the floor. If it takes less than 10 seconds, not enough weight was added. If you can't get your arm down after 20 seconds, too much weight was added. Ask the coach to adjust the amount of weight you receive.

7. When the coach removes his foot, take a deep breath and relax the arm. Un-Lock. Shake out the arm if you feel the need. First-timers usually need a Tiny Torque after each of these three stretches.

Return to the palm-up position, and get ready for two more stretches. (Aren't you feeling better already?)

What the Coach Does

1. Place the PIC's arm in the Forearm Up position, palm facing up and arm at a 30-degree angle from the body. If this hurts the PIC's elbow or shoulder, move the hand out farther so that the forearm bones remain parallel to the floor.

2. Curl up the toes of your Working foot and place it lightly straight down on the PIC's biceps, about 1 inch above the elbow. Don't let the biceps squish out to one side or the other.

3. Tell the PIC to bring her hand up and gently touch the back of your calf muscle (as in figure 10.13A). Now begin adding weight to the biceps until your PIC says "Stop!" Remember to ask, "Can you take a little more?" And remember, Coach, this is a tough stretch.

Hint: Because this stretch requires more work, the amount of weight you add may not be as much as in previous stretches.

4. Tell your PIC to Lock up.

5. Now tell the PIC to peel back her hand *slowly*, reaching with her fingertips for the floor. Start the 10-count as soon as the peeling motion begins. Make sure the PIC is moving very slowly, keeping the arm in

toward her body, not bending it outward. The closer the arm stays to the body, the better the stretch. The hand should be heading toward its original position on the floor (as in figure 10.13C).

Hint: Experience with the Bicep has shown that a lot of PICs take too much weight on this stretch. In order to allow a good stretch, you may have to cheat a little to help the PIC get her arm all the way down to the floor. Many times, the PIC will not be able to lower her arm completely because she took too much weight. If so, let up on the weight a tiny bit to keep the PIC's arm moving downward. If you don't ease up on weight, the PIC may get discouraged and quit stretching. The trick is to ease up on weight in tiny increments so the PIC doesn't know you're doing it. Got it? It should take about 10 seconds for the PIC to get her hand all the way to the mat. As you get better, the PIC won't even notice you cheated. It's more important to stretch the arm completely than it is to "win" as coach by refusing to let up on weight. Remember, this is a team effort.

---

6. Keep encouraging the PIC to peel her fingertips toward the floor, slowly, deliberately. The object is to lay the back of the hand and arm flat on the carpet or mat. When the fingertips reach the floor (as in figure 10.13D), keep encouraging the stretch until the wrist touches and flattens on the floor (as in figure 10.13E).

7. Cross-check: Make sure the PIC maintains the Lock, breathes, and keeps eyes open. This stretch may hurt, so keep the words of encouragement coming frequently!

8. Once the PIC's fingers and wrist are flat on the floor, remove your foot and immediately start a Tiny Torque. Tell the PIC to relax, take a breath, and Un-Lock. Then do a few more Tiny Torques, especially the first few times you do this stretch.

Repeat two more times, moving the foot 1/4-inch up the arm each time.

Stretch 4: Bicep Torque

This technique requires a little more finesse from the coach. The coach not only will be adding weight with the foot, she'll use the foot to catch and roll muscle over the PIC's upper arm and hold it there during the entire stretch.

This stretch requires a bit more of the coach's Working foot, so follow directions carefully. If the PIC is able to rotate and place the back of her hand on the floor at the end of the stretch, you haven't added weight correctly. Go back and try again. Know this: The PIC will whine when you add weight.

Coach, read the instructions carefully for signs you're doing this stretch correctly. If you're not, start over and try again. Remember, practice makes perfect. This is the most difficult technique to do, and it's the coach's job to get it right (or risk having some toes chomped on by the PIC!).

What the PIC Does

➤ Keep your pinky on the floor for this stretch.

➤ Keep breathing, and keep your eyes open.

1. Lie face up on the mat. Take a deep breath and relax.

2. Place your arm in the Forearm Down position, with palm facing down and the lower arm parallel to the rest of the body, as in figure 10.14A. The elbow should be slightly but noticeably bent.

3. The coach will place his foot on the outside of your upper arm and roll tissue and muscle over the bone, holding it in place while adding weight, as in figure 10.14B. Take as much weight as you can.

Hint: Be aware with this stretch. Your crazy bone at the elbow should not feel as if it's being zinged or in danger. If it buzzes or zings, tell the coach to readjust his weight or put a support under your arm or shoulder. See chapter 7 for tips about pads and supports.

---

4. When the coach instructs you, Lock up and maintain the Lock throughout the stretch.

5. After the coach adds weight and begins counting to 10, slowly spread out your fingers and rotate your hand so your palm is heading toward your body (as in figure 10.14C). The goal is to try to turn your hand over, rotating and leading with your thumb (think "hitchhiking"). Your hand should turn over first, then your wrists, then your forearm. Keep your fingers reaching out and apart, palm stretched out, and hand wide open. Leave your pinky on the floor; rotate and reach outward from the elbow. Your hand will not be able to turn all the way over; just rotate it as far as it will go and then hold that stretch (as in figure 10.14D). Do not curl your fingers—that's cheating.

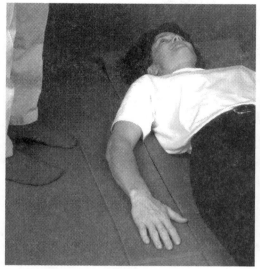

A   Forearm Down Position

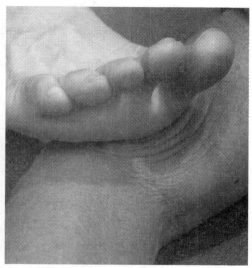

B   Adding Weight and Rolling the Flesh

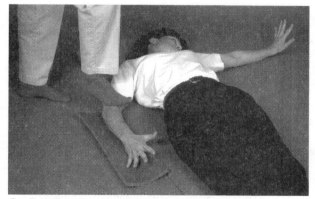

C   Rotating the Hand, Wrist, and Forearm

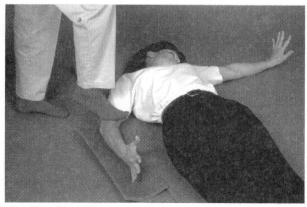

D   The Stretch

Figure 10.14   Bicep Torque

Hint: If the back of your hand is able to touch the floor, your coach doesn't have a good enough grip on your biceps muscle, so start over and try again. In a proper Bicep Torque, your hand should not turn over more than the woman's hand in figure 10.14D. If your hand turns all the way over, your coach didn't get a good enough grip. You'll have to try again.

6. At the end of a 10-count, the coach will remove his weight and ask you to relax. Un-Lock and shake out your arm if needed. Take a deep breath. Tell your coach if you need to rest or a Tiny Torque.

Now return to Forearm Down position and get ready for two more stretches.

What the Coach Does

Note: Do **not** use a stand for this stretch.

1. Place the PIC's arm in the Forearm Down position, with the forearm parallel to the body and the palm flat on the floor (as in figure 10.14A). The elbow should be slightly but noticeably bent.

2. In order to get the proper effect, your Base foot needs to be perpendicular to the PIC's forearm and about one foot away from her upper arm. By doing this first you assure yourself of getting the best and most powerful grip on the PIC's arm.

3. Flex the toes of your Working foot and place it about 1 inch above the PIC's elbow (as in figure 10.14B). Here's the tricky part: Add just enough weight for the ball of your foot to grab some fleshy tissue above the PIC's elbow joint. Roll the flesh and muscle over the upper-arm bone, and continue rolling it toward the center of the PIC's body. Roll it at a downward angle toward the PIC's chest. With the ball of the foot, hold the tissue as tightly as possible and keep it there. Keep your heel low. It will hurt the PIC, but it shouldn't feel as if you're pinching or crushing the upper-arm bone. You're positioning your foot as close to the bone as you can, but don't crush the bone. You've got to get near the bone to slide the flesh over it. This is simple, but not necessarily easy. Maintain the hold on the tissue when your PIC says "Stop!" or "Enough weight!"

Hint: Stay off the bone. You're looking for a spot right next to the bone, yet you should be able to feel the bone as you roll the tissue over it. Just don't push directly into the bone. I can't emphasize this enough: *Stay off the bone;* just feel it. This stretch is touchy and it might cause the PIC to wince a little (or a lot). It's too much weight if your PIC panics or hits your leg!

4. Ask your PIC to Lock. Make sure a good Lock is maintained during the entire stretch.

5. Begin counting to 10.

Hint: Count very slowly. This stretch takes a while for PICs to get accustomed to, and your 10-second count should reflect this.

Your PIC will slowly rotate her hand over, keeping the pinky finger on the floor and leading over with the thumb. It's like hitchhiking with the thumb, with the hand glued to the floor at the pinky. Fingers should be straight, palm stretched out, and the hand opened wide. Do not the let the PIC curl the fingers. If the thumb ends pointing straight up, bingo! That's the correct stretch! If the PIC says "Ouch!" at the beginning of the outward hand rotation and is unable to move, you've got the perfect stretch going! Keep it up! (Remember, this shouldn't be easy for the PIC to do.) Encourage the PIC to play with that position, going after the pain by stretching and rotating as far as possible.

Hint: The PIC should not be able to lay the back of her hand flat on the floor at the end of the stretch. If she does, you didn't get a good enough grasp of the upper-arm tissue when you added weight. Go back and try again. The PIC should feel as if she's trying to turn the hand over completely, but she shouldn't actually be able to accomplish it. She should be "ouching" and stretching the hand more than she is actually flattening it. That's the sign of an effective stretch. Here's another sign: The PIC will swear you're peeling the hide right off her arm, but when it's over, she says, "Oh, wow! That's much looser! Do it again." That's a sign of a great Bicep Torque.

A gender-related tip: Experience with this stretch has shown that men almost always will try to rotate outward from the shoulder. Rotating should start with the hand and should occur only below the elbow. This is an elbow technique, not a shoulder technique, and that's an important point to remember. If the PIC moves the shoulder, stop and start again. A finely executed Bicep Torque will get rid of most elbow problems. A poor technique just hurts.

If the PIC whines and says she did the best she could, say this: "Okay, let's start again. This time, roll your hand over but start only with the fingers doing the rolling, then the hand. Keep the fingers straight. Roll over the wrist to the elbow. It will feel completely different than the last time. It should hurt worse, but better. You will feel a nasty pull in your elbow."

6. Cross-check: Make sure the PIC maintains a good Lock throughout the stretch.

7. At the end of a 10-count, remove your foot and tell the PIC to breathe. This is a hard stretch, so give your PIC time to relax and give her a Tiny Torque if needed. If this is the PIC's first time doing the Bicep Torque, she'll need it.

To complete a Bicep Torque set, repeat two more times, moving the foot 1/4-inch up or down the arm each time. If you started with your foot too high on the PIC's arm for the first stretch, it's okay to do another stretch closer to the elbow. Proximity to the elbow is the key to this stretch's effectiveness. How can you tell if you're close enough? At the end of three well executed stretches, pain in the elbow should be gone.

Stretch 5: Hole in the Shoulder

The nickname for this technique is "reaching and screeching." It is the most powerful stretch to relieve pain in your upper back, neck, or inside of the shoulder joint.

You may be thinking, "Hole in the shoulder? Isn't that your armpit?" No, the hole in your shoulder is not your armpit. On the front of your shoulder, just below the shoulder joint, you'll find a natural indentation in your body. It's well below the collar bone and slightly toward the armpit. It's just before a ridge of muscle that goes into your armpit. See it? Feel it. Stick the fingers of your opposite hand into it to find it. Let your arm hang down, relaxed. The "hole" is shaped like an inverted and slightly slanted *V*. It's the fleshy part, not the bony part.

It is important to understand that this is not on the breast. Make sure you have the right area or you'll create a buzz in your arm. With Hole in the Shoulder, the coach will place her heel—not the arch of the foot—into that hole and direct a series of powerful stretches.

Hint: When the PIC is a woman, the coach must be careful not to step on her breast!

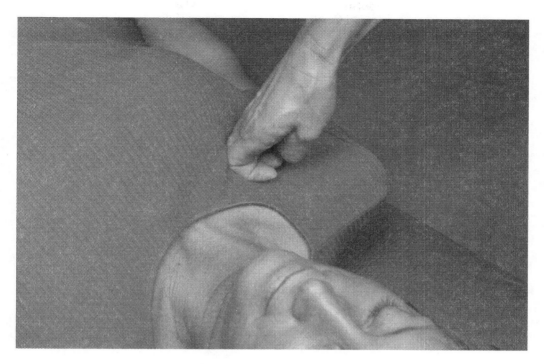

Figure 10.15 Find the Hole in Your Shoulder

What the PIC Does

1. Lie flat on the floor, both hands relaxed and straight down at your sides in a Forearm Up position. (When you Lock during this stretch, you will do so only with your feet, head, and neck, not with the opposite arm.)

2. Before the coach adds weight, practice the three movements you will make with each stretch:

   ▶ With the first stretch (figure 10.16) you will sweep both arms—palms up—along the floor from your sides until both are straight out from your shoulders. You'll look like a giant capital T. (It's like making a snow angel very slowly.) Do not move your arms higher than your shoulders.

   ▶ During the second stretch, do the same sweeping motion along the floor with the palms down (figure 10.17).

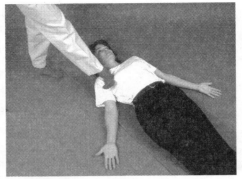

A   Beginning

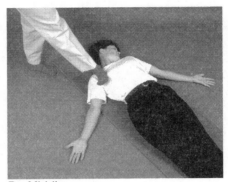

B   Middle

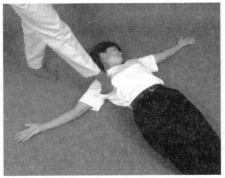

C   End

Figure 10.16   Hole in the Shoulder: Palms Up

> ► During the third stretch (figure 10.18), do the same sweeping motion with the thumbs up and the pinky fingers on the floor; the hand should be flat and perpendicular to the floor. This is called the Pinky Drag. (Cute, eh?)

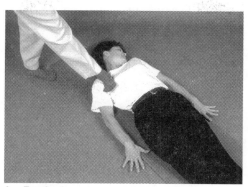

A   Beginning

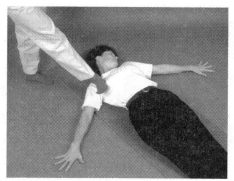

B   Middle

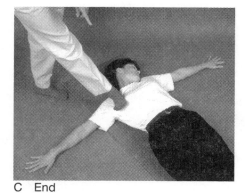

C   End

Figure 10.17   Hole in the Shoulder: Palms Down

3. Take a deep breath and relax. Remember, arms are at your sides, palms up.

4. The coach will take her heel and place it in the hole in your shoulder. If it doesn't feel comfortable to you, or if it hits bone or breast tissue,

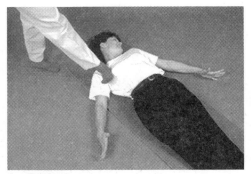

A   Beginning

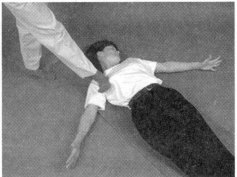

B   Middle

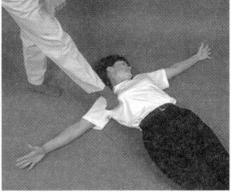

C   End

Figure 10.18   Hole in the Shoulder: Pinky Drag

grasp your coach's heel with your opposite hand and move it around
until it's firmly in the shoulder's hole. Move it around a few times, if
necessary, and you'll eventually feel the right place. It will be tender
but fleshy. You'll feel a natural "hole" in that area. Do not let the

coach put a heel next to the collar bone—that is *not* the hole. Remember, it's fleshy.

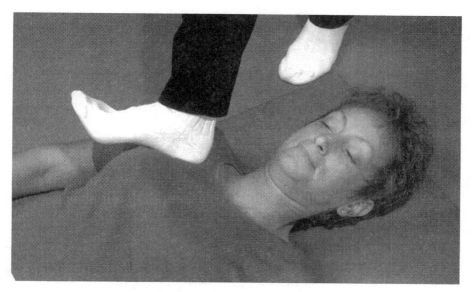

Figure 10.19   Hole in the Shoulder Heel Placement

5. The coach will add weight with her heel until you say stop.

Hint: If your body is tensed/tight or if you're holding your breath, the heel will be prevented from moving into the hole as far as it can. Relax. Breathe deeply. Relax again. Now relax your butt. Consciously loosen your shoulders and upper body several times and allow the heel to slide in as far it can. Take as much weight as you can.

---

6. When the coach tells you to Lock, keep your arms at your sides. Flex your toes toward your head, with your heels pushing away from your butt, and slowly roll your head away from the coach with your nose pointing down toward your shoulder, as in figure 10.20. Maintain this modified Lock during the entire stretch.

7. When the coach tells you to begin, make sure that the area under the coach's heel is taut. Then, slowly and simultaneously sweep both your arms along the floor, upward toward your upper body. Keep your palms up. Move *very slowly*, reaching outward with your arms and hands as far as you can. Keep the shoulder area relaxed. Keep

elbows almost locked and wrists straight. Pay attention to how each arm feels, and stretch each arm as both arms move.

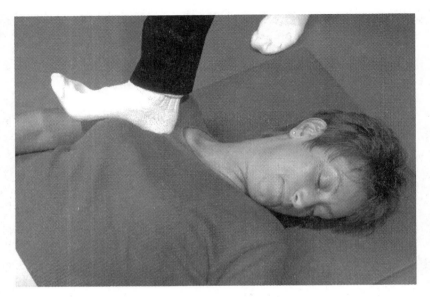

Figure 10.20   Head Turn

Hint: Your arms may feel different; one may pull or hurt more than the other. Go for the pain and pull it out!

You are stretching your entire body, so make sure you bring up both hands simultaneously. The middle of this position (as in figure 10.16B, 10.17B, and 10.18B) is a good place to stop, relax, breathe, and begin again. This mid-stretch stop is optional, but it enhances the power of the stretch (and can ease upper-back pain).

8. Keep breathing! It's likely you'll tense up and hold your breath or close your eyes. Don't! Keep your eyes open and lungs working! Always try to breathe under the coach's foot. Proper breathing produces a better stretch.

9. When your arms are at a 90-degree angle from the trunk of your body, the coach will call the stretch over. Take a deep breath into the area where the coach's foot is and let out the breath with gusto as the coach removes her heel. Return your arms to your sides. Shake them out or roll your shoulders if you feel the need.

Hint: Turning the hands over and taking a deep breath at the same time is the best way to end all Hole in the Shoulder techniques (as in figure 10.21). A beginner may not be able to do this, but try to work up to it. This is especially helpful for upper back pain and headaches.

Get ready to do the stretch two more times—once with palms facing down, and once with your pinky fingers touching the floor.

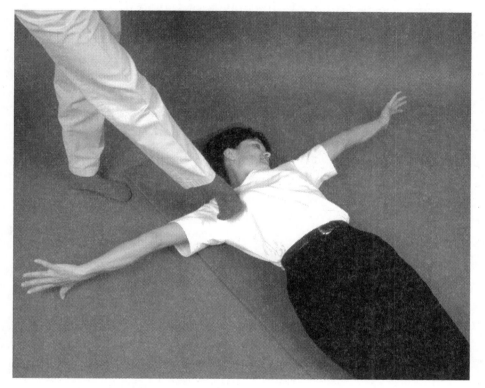

Figure 10.21   The Best Ending

What the Coach Does

Reminders:

▶ With Hole in the Shoulder, your *heel* applies weight.

▶ Where you stand is the most important part of this whole technique. It's possible to stand in the wrong place, so pay close attention. Stand above the PIC's head, out and a bit away from the shoulder being stretched. You will be standing 6–12 inches above the PIC, on the same side of the body being stretched. Remember: Same foot, same side. If you're stretching the PIC's right side, use your right foot and stand on the PIC's right side. Place your right arm on a chair behind you and to your right.

When you are truly in the shoulder's "hole," your leg should feel no strain. Your foot/heel should feel as if it's gone straight into a natural depression or spot and stopped there. If holding the heel in place is difficult, strains your groin area, or strains your butt, you are either standing too close to the PIC or not standing far enough to the PIC's side for this technique. Your stance for this stretch should feel easy; if it's not, you are doing something wrong. Stop, remove your heel, readjust your Base foot, and start again.

Try to get the angle right the first few times. It'll keep you and your PIC from suffering. If you place the foot wrong, you'll use pressure, not weight, and the person on the floor will get sore. With practice, you'll get the feel for the proper angle and position of the heel.

1. Position your PIC on the mat so that both arms are down at his sides, palms up.

2. Before you start, ask your PIC to practice the three sweeping motions for this stretch.
   - During the first stretch (figure 10.16), tell the PIC to sweep the hands up from the side of the body along the floor, both palms up. After the stretch, both arms return to the sides.
   - During the second stretch (figure 10.17), ask the PIC to do the same sweeping motion with palms down.
   - During the third stretch (figure 10.18), ask the PIC to do the same sweeping motion with the thumbs pointed up, pinky fingers on the floor. This is called Pinky Drag.

3. Take your heel and place it into the hole in your PIC's shoulder. You may have to move the heel around a few times (gently!) to find the hole.

Hint: If you're having a problem finding the spot, try this: Ask the PIC to put his left hand in his right armpit (or vice versa), with the thumb sticking out on top, just below the front of his shoulder. Where the first knuckle of the thumb rests is the "hole." Place your heel there and feel the indentation. Allow your heel to find the lowest spot, just above the armpit, without falling out of the hole. Never push the foot against any breast tissue! If you hit bone, you're also in the wrong spot. Look for soft tissue and keep looking till you find it. If necessary, ask the PIC to grasp your heel and position it for you.

---

4. Point your toes outward, away from the PIC's body, as in figure 10.22. This is a safety issue. If you were to fall, you don't want to fall on your partner, and your partner isn't keen about the idea, either. Your knee should lock, just as the PIC's feet Lock. If your heel tries to slip out of the hole, reposition the Base foot above the PIC's shoulder and place your heel again until it feels right.

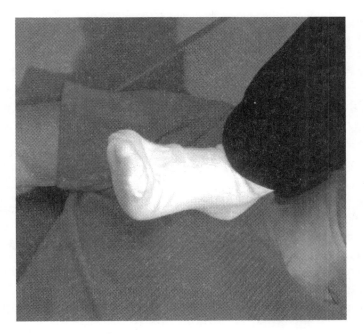

Figure 10.22 Toes Up and Out

5. Apply weight straight—not sideways—into the PIC's hole in the shoulder. If you feel resistance or tightness, ask the PIC to take a deep breath, relax the shoulders and upper body, and relax the butt. You'll feel your heel slip deeper and more comfortably into the hole. You may have to encourage the PIC to relax several times before you feel the entire shoulder area loosen and allow your foot into the hole. When the PIC says "Stop!" hold the heel in place.

6. Ask the PIC to Lock, but make sure he keeps his arms by his sides.

7. Now tell the PIC to *slowly* sweep both arms, palms up, along the floor until they are perpendicular with the trunk of the body. Elbows should be locked, wrists straight, arms and hands reaching out as far as they can. Remind your PIC to keep breathing and keep eyes open! It's possible that one arm will move easier or quicker than the other. Praise the good arm, encourage the slower arm. (For example: "Your

right arm's coming fine, keep working on the left! Pull! Stretch! A few more inches! Keep reaching!") Do not allow the arms to move beyond being perpendicular with the shoulder.

8. Cross-check: Make sure the head-shoulder-foot Lock remains in place during the stretch. You'll have a lot to check while watching, so keep a watchful eye on the PIC. Keep a special eye on the head, because it tends to return to the center. Make sure it stays over toward the shoulder.

9. When the PIC's arms form a giant capital T with the body, tell him to take a deep breath into the area where your foot is. Make sure the arms are up and even before asking for the breath. Then ask for an exhale. As the PIC exhales, your heel will naturally leave the hole in the shoulder. Lift out your heel and call the stretch over. The PIC should return his arms to the sides of his body.

10. Relax, take a breath and encourage your PIC to do the same.

Get ready to complete a Hole in the Shoulder set, by repeating two more times, once with palms down, and once with pinky fingers dragging on the floor. Each time, move the angle of the heel by repositioning the heel of the Base foot about 1/8-inch to 1/4-inch.

Now, to continue stretching, move to the PIC's opposite side and repeat all of the stretches you've done: Forearm Up, Forearm Down, Bicep, Bicep Torque, and Hole in the Shoulder. Remember to use Tiny Torque and Mr. Twister as needed for stinging or lingering pain.

After you've stretched both sides, it's time for the last stretch, the Traps. Remember, the Traps are only done *after* the PIC's right and left sides have been through the first five stretches.

Stretch 6: The Traps

Traps is short for trapezius, the muscle that drapes and connects the shoulder, neck, and head. This stretch is the frosting on all the Rossiter techniques. It will be everyone's favorite because the looseness and freedom of movement it produces are so noticeable and quick.

If you overdo this stretch, it will cause a sore back, sore neck, or bad headache, so use it prudently and *only* after doing at least the Hole in the Shoulder stretch first.

The Traps is done after the first five stretches have been completed on both sides of the PIC's body—Forearm Up through Hole in the Shoulder. It is done with the PIC seated in a straight-backed chair. This is the final upper body stretch, and this is the fun one.

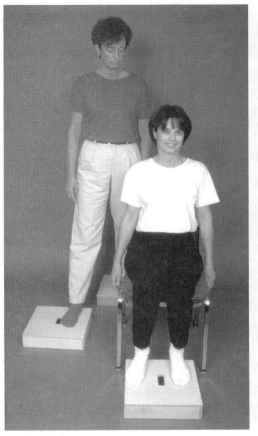

A   Beginning

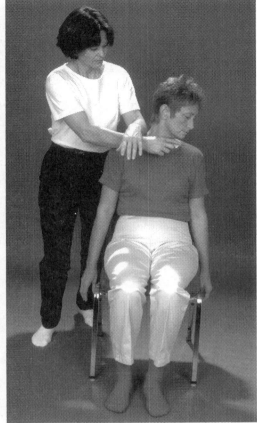

B   Moving the Head

Figure 10.23   The Traps

Reminders for PIC and coach:

► The Traps is done with the PIC seated in a straight chair (preferably a chair with no arms) and the Coach standing next to and slightly behind the PIC.

► The coach will use his elbow to apply weight. No feet or heels are involved.

What the PIC Does

1. Sit up straight in a straight-backed chair, preferably a chair with no arms (as in figure 10.23A). Place your feet flat on the floor (use a phone book or pads if you need to). Move your butt up against the

back of the chair. No slouching! Hang your shoulders and arms loosely at your sides. Doing so makes the techniques easier for you and your coach. If you don't sit up straight, your back will get sore.

Hint: There are two ways to do the Traps. You can let both arms hang relaxed and down at the sides, or you can reach down with both arms at the sides during the stretch to increase its effectiveness. Reaching adds power to this stretch. Reaching also may be necessary for bigger and bulkier PICs because the coach will not be able to apply enough weight if the PIC's arms are loose.

---

2. Your coach will place his opposite-side elbow into your shoulder and apply gentle weight straight down into the fleshly part of the top of your shoulder. Say "Stop!" when it's enough weight. The coach's hand will hang loosely in front of you if he's doing it right.

3. After weight has been applied, your coach will tell you to gently pivot your head slowly away from him. Let your head angle down toward the floor as it moves away. Turn as far toward your shoulder as you can. This will hurt pleasantly!

4. When your head is at its farthest point away from the coach, slowly move it down toward the floor, leading with your nose (as in figure 10.23B). Move the nose downward as far as you can. Feel the stretch in your shoulders, up into your neck, and into your head and face. While you're stretching with your head, reach your hands toward the floor as well. Your shoulders should shift downward, not up, when you reach. Do not slouch. Now slowly bring the head back up so your chin is parallel with the floor. Slowly, move your head down toward the floor a second time.

Hint: If you find a place that's particularly painful, move your head up and down *slowly* in that area and consciously work it out. Don't tilt the nose upward when going after painful areas. If the nose points too high, you'll pinch your neck. If you'd like, you can pivot your head downward a third time; if possible, turn it even farther away from the coach before moving it downward. Doing so makes the stretch more powerful, especially if you're reaching down with your hands.

---

5. Your coach will instruct you on when and how to bring your head back to its starting center position and declare the stretch over. Take a deep breath and relax.

6. Wiggle your shoulders up and down a bit if you feel the need, and get ready to complete the Traps.

What the Coach Does

Reminders: Your stance and ability to add weight with your elbow are important to the success of the Traps, so read these tips carefully before you start.

▸ If you're stretching the PIC's left side, you'll use your right elbow to add weight. Left shoulder, right elbow. Got that? This is the only exception to the same side–same foot rule.

▸ Use the area as close to the tip of the elbow as possible (figure 10.24), but *don't* use just the tip.

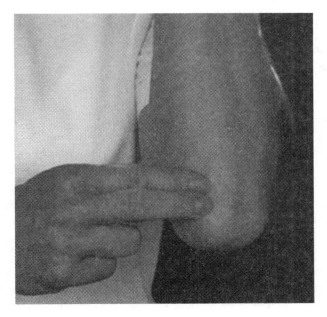

Figure 10.24 Traps Elbow

▸ Get your feet in position. If you're stretching the PIC's right side, place your left foot at least 12 inches behind the PIC's back. Your foot should be pointing toward the PIC's neck. Place your right foot next to and below the PIC's shoulder, the one about to be stretched. Notice the coach's feet in figure 10.25. Make sure that your back foot isn't sideways.

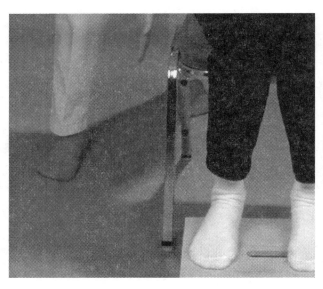

Figure 10.25   Foot Position

- Bend your knees slightly. Relax your shoulders (they have no set position). Bend your working elbow to a 90-degree angle; it's the best angle from which to add weight.

- Apply weight with your working elbow. To find the proper place on your elbow, place your middle finger on the tip of your elbow. Now place your first finger 1-inch from the tip of your elbow onto your forearm. That 1-inch flat area next to the tip of your elbow is the spot you'll use to add weight into your PIC's shoulder. Memorize this spot. Do not add weight from farther forward on your forearm (away from the elbow) or with just the tip of the elbow; doing so will cause pain in the coach's shoulders.

- When adding weight, keep your forearm parallel to the floor. Your hand should not be up in the air. It should be in front of and to the side of your PIC's face, no higher and absolutely relaxed. Your hand should droop.

- Because this stretch is different from the others, the coach has what could be considered a Lock position while adding weight. Paying attention to all of the reminders automatically leads to this Lock position. It's basically like this: Your body should Lock with your shoulders down and relaxed on your rib cage. Don't bend or lean with the shoulders, just keep the shoulders straight and in line with your torso. If your shoulders creep up during this technique, you're likely to end up with a sore neck, headache, or both.

► The trick to applying weight is to bend your knees and allow your body—not your shoulder or shoulder muscles—to give the weight from that 1-inch flat spot starting at your elbow. If you keep your shoulders straight and in position resting in line with your rib cage, bend your knees, and settle gently into the PIC's shoulder with your flattened elbow, you will automatically add weight.

Let me say that again: Bending your knees slowly and evenly adds weight. There's no upper-body pushing or leaning required. Keep your back straight. Stick out your butt as you bend your knees. If your butt doesn't stick out, you're not doing adding weight correctly and the technique won't work.

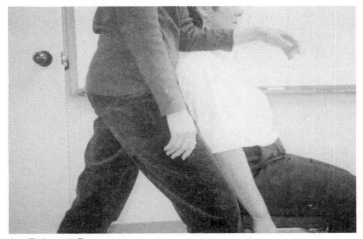

A   Relaxed Butt

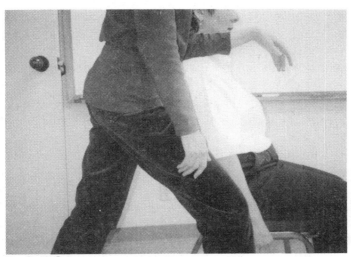

B   Butt Out

Figure 10.26   Knee Position

This stance may take a few practices to get it right, so make sure you're comfortable. Once you understand the stance and how to add weight, begin the stretch. An easy way to see if you're doing this technique right is to face a mirror. If you see your shoulders creep up, stop and start again. If you don't learn the stance properly, you'll get sore.

Okay. Ready to start?

1. Make sure your PIC is seated in a straight-backed chair, arms and shoulders hanging loosely at her sides. The PIC's butt should be against the back of the chair and the PIC's feet should be flat on the floor. Prop up the feet with phone books or pads, if necessary. Do not allow the PIC to slouch.

2. Stand next to the PIC as described. If you're adding weight with your right elbow, place your right foot (knee slightly bent) behind the PIC and your left foot next to the chair with your knee straight (see figure 10.25). Remember the spot to use on your elbow? Place the elbow straight down and flatly into the PIC's shoulder, not into the neck. Get into the fleshy part of the shoulder. Feel around till you find the right spot. Ask, "Can you take a little more weight?" until the PIC says "Stop!" Go for the gold!

Hint: When adding weight, allow your body to move down onto the PIC's shoulder. Do not bend your body or lean sideways from the waist into your PIC to add weight, or you'll begin hurting, too. Keep your front knee bending forward; bend your back leg slightly as you move into the shoulder. Remember, stick out your butt.

---

3. When weight is applied, begin counting to 10 and use your other hand to guide and tell the PIC to turn her head *slowly* away from you, keeping her chin parallel to the floor as her head slowly turns. When the PIC's head is turned as far as it can toward the shoulder, use your fingers to point and direct her head slowly downward, reaching with the nose toward the shoulder and floor (see figure 10.27). Then direct the PIC's head back up until the chin is again parallel with the floor. *This is all done very slowly.*

Hint: You may feel knots in the PIC's shoulder moving back and forth under your elbow. Encourage the PIC to nod *slowly* up and down into those knotted areas to work them out. Let the PIC stay in these knotty places and unkink them for whatever amount of time feels comfortable.

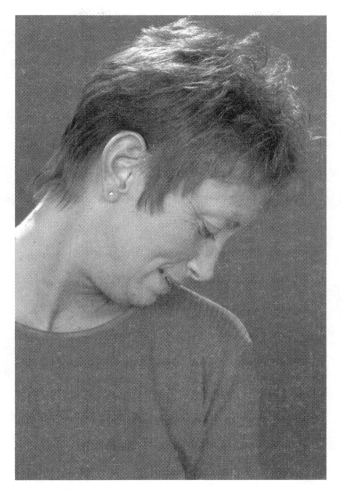

Figure 10.27   Nose to Shoulder

4. During the stretch, make sure the PIC reaches with her hands down toward the floor. Give an incentive, such as "Reach for that $100 bill on the floor!" If the PIC's hands are reaching, the upper-body stretch is far more effective. Both sides need to be reaching simultaneously for the floor.

5. When the 10-count is over, remove your elbow and tell your PIC to take a deep breath and relax. Have the PIC shrug and rotate both shoulders, as in figure 10.28, to test the new freedom of movement.

To complete the Traps set, repeat it two more times and reposition your elbow a little differently each time in the fleshy part of the shoulder. Find the icky, awful places. Then do three stretches on the PIC's other shoulder.

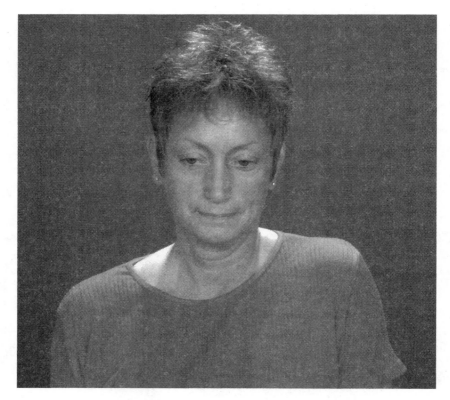

Figure 10.28   Shoulder Shrug

Congratulations! You've just completed the first series of upper-body stretches using the Rossiter System. Don't you feel better? Didn't I tell you this would make you feel lighter, freer, and less achy?

Don't forget to use Tiny Torques and Mr. Twisters whenever you need them!

The Rossiter Dessert: Once you've completed Rossiter stretches on both sides, the best thing you can do is go for a walk. Walking is the ideal exercise to help connective tissue stay supple and stretched out and to help it return to its normal state. Walk with a purpose. Walk as if you're going somewhere. Walk with a friend. Walk for fun. And remember to wear good, supportive walking shoes.

If you're interested in stretches for the lower back, go to chapters 11–13.

Chapter 11

"Oh, My Achin' Back. . . .": The Rossiter System and Back Pain

When you think about it, the back has an incredible job to do. It keeps the body upright. It allows the body to bend, tilt, twist, crouch, swivel, turn, walk, run, sit, squat, stoop, and poop.

This may seem truly odd, but all the Rossiter stretches to relieve pain and tightness in the lower back are done on the front of the thigh. That's right—the front of the thigh. None of the back stretches involves touching anyone's back. (You can relax now. No one will step on your back!) These back stretches have an unusual evolution, a melting-pot existence of childhood encounters with *National Geographic* magazines, a bike-race experiment with human thighs, and some light-bulb observations of people's bodies that have helped me conceive of the TBS (Tummy-Butt-Shoulders) concept (or its alter ego, Tight Butt Syndrome). Somehow, this chapter will attempt to make sense of these topics and more.

Join the Back Pain Crowd

Because it has so many things to do, the back is an extremely vulnerable part of the body, which is one of the reasons back pain is so common. Experts estimate that in the United States, eight in ten people suffer back pain at some time in life, and about 5 percent of the population has chronic back pain. According to the National Center for Health Statistics, back pain is the second leading reason (behind common colds) why Americans visit their doctors. It's also responsible for about $15 billion in medical bills and lost wages a year, according to the American Academy of Orthopaedic Surgeons (1999).

The Rossiter System classifies back pain as either Type One or Type Two, and both types will be explained later in the chapter.

It's important to know from the start, however, that when you begin doing the back stretches, you may need to adjust the techniques in the middle of a workout, based on the type of pain you're dealing with.

All the stretches start the same, but once you've determined if you have Type One or Type Two pain, you can quickly alter your techniques to accommodate the specific pain type and make the stretches their most effective. (Read the tips and precautions in the next chapter before you begin the actual stretches.)

Nine out of ten times, the techniques will be done as described, because most people have Type Two back pain. The stretches are based on the assumption that you have Type Two back pain. However, you'll also learn about the symptoms that indicate Type One pain, which means you'll have to switch to the PIC's other side to do the stretches. Trust me, it'll get clearer as you read on.

You may be eager to start the stretches immediately, but it helps to understand the anatomy and philosophy of the stretches. So, let's look first at why and how the back and the Rossiter back stretches work. If you skip this information now, you'll be back. These are simple concepts, but it helps to have the basics.

The Evolution of the Rossiter System Back Program

As a child or teenager, did you ever occasionally leaf through your parents' copies of *National Geographic* for, shall we say, the natural beauty? I did. (Back then I had hormones and hair. Now I lust for Viagra and Rogaine.)

If you were to go back today and gawk at those photographs of naked humans in primitive societies, you'd notice one thing (well, besides the nakedness). When the people in those photos stand upright, they don't hold in their stomachs. They live and thrive in societies untouched by modern culture ("Suck in that gut, Mr. Macho!") and modern fashion ("Squeeze into those skin-tight jeans, Ms. Glamour"). Bellies were designed to be relaxed, and the *National Geographic* bellies are indeed relaxed. They're out there. They're noticeable. Some are like bowls of jelly. They're comfortable. They're natural-looking—and probably not causing back pain.

Now, let's compare those relaxed, natural bellies with life in the United States. (This requires your participation.)

First, stand up. Once you're up, relax as many muscles in your body as possible. Feel how your body naturally gives way to something more comfortable? Good. Tighten again, and then relax the same muscles again. Got the feeling?

Okay, here's the test: From a relaxed position, slowly tighten your stomach muscles. Did you feel the stomach tighten? Good. Now relax the stomach muscles and then tighten them again. This time, notice that your butt—even more specifically, your butt hole—tightens, too. Isn't this interesting? (If you cheated and did this exercise while sitting, you'll notice that it worked anyway.) Why does this happen?

Before explaining further, let's try the reverse. Remain standing and relax all your muscles again. Now tighten that little butt hole of yours and notice what happens. Your stomach tightens, too. Why? They're connected. You cannot purposely tighten one without the other, because the stomach and butt naturally tighten and relax simultaneously.

Here's another test: Tighten your tummy again and notice what happens to your shoulders. Did you feel them shift back or drop a bit? Relax again, and then tighten your shoulders (to the way you think you should look), noticing what happens to your tummy and butt. Did you feel them tighten? What a connection! No matter which one you tighten, the other two tighten and shift automatically. I call this connection TBS, short for tummy-butt-shoulders. Over the years, my trainers have given it a different moniker: tight butt syndrome.

If you live in the good ol' US-of-A, you probably have TBS. It's cultural, and it's spreading. It's a result of vanity and expectations. It's what happens when you don't want to buy the next-size slacks or skirt, even though what you're wearing now is too tight.

Instead of buying clothes that fit comfortably, what do you do? You hold in your stomach. You suck it in as far as is temporarily comfortable and tell yourself it looks good. Again, it's cultural, part of that svelte look people try to achieve—the one that defies most basic principles of human anatomy. With nearly one-third of the U.S. population now classified as overweight, this self-imposed tension makes a lot of people look as though they've been poured into their clothes.

Let me give you an example: One year, I worked with a tiny, ninety-year-old woman in my Rolfing practice. She suffered from back pain. She had a striking resemblance to a pale prune that had been lost under a bed for a few years. She wore thick makeup. On a really tall day, she was all of four-foot-eight, and she had bright red hair (at least on some parts of her hair; the other parts were white).

She was standing in my office in 1920-era underwear and a slip. The underwear drooped to her calves and the slip hung at her knees. It looked as if the underwear waistband were tucked somewhere up under her breasts.

"Are you holding in your tummy?" I asked innocently.

"Absolutely not," she said firmly.

As I talked with her, I gently and reassuringly told her it was okay to let her tummy relax, to let loose, to let it all hang out. And finally with a big sigh, she let it go.

"How does your back feel now?" I asked.

"It feels good," she said, somewhat astonished. "There's no pain." Then she suddenly looked at me with that cross-old-woman look and sucked her stomach back in. "But it looks awful," she said, and she steadfastly refused to let her stomach muscles relax. She still wanted her back pain "fixed," just not that way.

TBS: It's Pervasive

The woman's experience, unfortunately, is the norm today for people of every age, height, and weight. They wear tight pants. They notch their belts beyond comfortable to make their waists look trimmer. If they wore a size 10 (or 42 regular) in 1969, by cracky, they'll be a size 10 (or 42 regular) today, too, even if they have to squeeze and hold their breath and lie down flat on the bed to get the zipper up. Sound familiar? Some women look as if their clothes are cutting them in half. Some men's belts are simply lost from view.

Even people who are trim and fit do it. Overweight, grossly overweight, obese, and morbidly obese people may try to hold in their stomachs, even though it's not apparent they're doing it. They may swear they're not holding anything in, but they've usually been doing it for so long that they can't tell. What they will admit is that their backs hurt, and that's the key to knowing they're tummy-suckers.

Many of the clients of my Rolfing practice had back problems. Usually, the onset of their back pain coincided with weight gain, wearing clothes that no longer fit comfortably, or donning high-heeled shoes—all sorts of factors that could be fixed or prevented. The clients were unaware of how tightly they held in their stomachs. To help them feel this tightness, I'd usually start a little in-office exercise after they'd recited a list of symptoms of what hurt and where. I didn't tell them this was for the back.

I'd look down at the client's belly, smile up at his or her face, and begin talking. Gradually, I'd shift my gaze away from the person's face and speak directly to the tummy. I'd start up a constant chatter: "Come on, come on, you can let go. Come on, baby! You can let go. Don't pay attention to that person up there [the client], just let that stomach relax. Come on, let go! Let go! Let go! You have my permission to let go!"

It always made people laugh, and I'd keep up the chatter—without being too personal—until something happened. And something always happened.

At some point in all that talk, I'd start to see a little quiver near the waist line. Then a bigger one, followed by a little droop. Then a bigger quiver. Then I'd get my face right next to the person's stomach and start again: "Come on, you can let go! You can let that stomach relax!" Finally, little by little, the stomach would relax and loosen up. And when the client finally let everything hang, I'd ask, "How does your back feel?" And every single one would say the same thing: the back pain was gone.

I learned two things: First, my clients wanted the right to a pain-free back without doing the necessary work. Second, modern-day culture glorifies flat stomachs, or else people wouldn't be so stubborn about sucking in their guts.

The problem is that when you tighten and flatten your tummy, your butt puckers. Quite simply, that means your back tightens. It's part of the body's balancing act, like a teeter-totter. When you tighten one part, the other part tightens, too. If you didn't, you'd tip over.

Part of that balancing act has to do with how the body puts on and stores weight. As people eat, the body's genius is that it knows exactly where to store and keep extra weight to minimize stress on the body. Whether you put on too many pounds or just the right amount of pounds, the body knows where to put it evenly and in a balanced way.

Let's say you eat a piece of cheesecake. The body distributes the cheesecake throughout the body to balance the weight, front to back and right to left. If you put on excess weight, the body still stands upright—it doesn't cave in or tip over, because the body doles out new weight evenly to both sides. Next time you're at the mall, observe people's bodies. If they're overweight, they're overweight on both sides of their bodies, aren't they? They're not just fat in one leg or all on one side of the waist. If they have large arms, the largeness involves both arms. If they're large-breasted, both breasts are oversized, not just the right or just the left. If they have heavy thighs, both thighs carry the weight, not one or the other. Big tummies are usually followed by big butts. The body always tries to be balanced.

Some imbalance is natural; some is artificial. When you see a svelte woman with a slender waist, tiny butt, and large breasts there's a chance she may be "artificially enhanced." That means fake breasts, or breast implants. Other women are just naturally big-breasted. The breasts don't appear to "fit" the rest of the body. In my Rolfing practice, women with large breasts often reported, "My upper back aches between my shoulder blades all the time, and I don't know why." Here's why: The upper body was designed for smaller breasts. To stay balanced with larger breasts, women need to tip back a little or pull back the shoulders, and they usually do both. Either or both eventually can cause headaches, migraines, back pains—all kinds of pain. Breast implants can cause other problems (beyond those women report from silicone). Some report chest pain or tightening across the chest. These are all examples of how the body initiates its own autobalancing system in response to any change, stress, or added weight.

Other imbalances occur because of how we live in our bodies. We create imbalances side to side. We always hold our babies on our left hip, leaving our right hand free. We work at a poorly designed work station that forces one side of the body to work harder than the other, or we do work that cannot be done any other way. Right-handed pitchers, welders, artists, and computer-mouse users know the sensation.

Over time, the person's muscles change and adapt to become more suited to the task, in effect changing the person's mass and power. Often, these imbalances and power shifts create pain.

The Muscular Balancing Act

The same balancing act happens in the body when muscles are tensed, strained, or overused. When you tighten one set of muscles in one location, the body's autobalancing system corrects the imbalance immediately by tightening somewhere else, usually with pain or discomfort. It happens every time you flex, move, or tense your arms, legs, back, stomach, or shoulders. And when you suck in your gut, you automatically tense your back, shoulders, and butt. That kind of balancing and shifting goes on all the time all over your body.

If you can tighten your stomach separately from your butt, you'll notice that you tilt forward. Your toes will push into the floor. Then you'll compensate by rolling the shoulders backward and tightening your butt. If won't be a grip-tight sensation—just enough to tense your back and to balance you upright again.

And if you tense and suck in all day long, you'll have tension all day (and eventually at night). This chronic tension also produces headaches, neck pain, shoulder aches, arm pain, even sinus headaches. Eventually, your conscious tightening will be balanced by unconscious tightening somewhere else. It will become a physical habit, and your body eventually will complain with pain. Remember, your body has to tell you when it's tired or hurting because it's designed that way. You can't alter the original design or intent.

But back pain is often the worst bugaboo. If you unconsciously (or consciously) tighten or tense your tummy, butt, or shoulders, you most likely will have back pain all day. Early on, it will occur in late afternoon and early evening.

Do you get back pain late in the day or after you eat? Do you get back pain as soon as you hike up your pants and hook your belt? Do you feel fine in bed but notice that nagging back pain starts about ten minutes after you get up and start moving?

Each of these phenomena are about the amount of space your body has in which to function, just as TBS is about space. If your body doesn't have enough internal space, it tells you. It may tell you immediately, it may tell you several hours later. If you're paying too much attention to how you look, you may be missing other important signals that your body is sending you about how it feels—signals about pain, the onset of disease, your tissue's need for nutrients and oxygen, and your tissue's need to move, hang loose, and be free.

If you're in pain because of TBS, you're also drawing energy away from your most valuable assets—your own personal satisfaction and your family. When you're in pain, you forget. You don't care. You're self-absorbed. So tummy-butt-shoulders, or tight butt syndrome, is painful in more ways than one.

And the next time you hear a coworker or friend complain about a sore or stiff neck, you already know what's going on. That little butt hole of theirs is tight, tight, tight.

From TBS to Thighs: The Cyclist Connection

In the late 1980s, I volunteered to provide Rolfing therapy to cyclists at a Multiple Sclerosis Society 150-mile bicycle race and fund-raiser. Cyclists stopped at checkpoints along the route complaining of cramps in their calves, pulled hamstrings, shin splints, and backaches. My job was to meet them at these stops and do mini-sessions of Rolfing.

I would work on or near the spots that hurt, send them on their way, and then meet up with them at the next checkpoint to do it again. Frequently, the same riders complained of the same aches and pains by the time they arrived at the next stop.

So I decided to try something different. I knew I had the ideal situation at this bike race—a group of people doing the same activity, all in the same basic physical shape, eating the same foods, and complaining of the same pains. It was like a perfect scientific mini-experiment.

As I thought about a good starting point for this experiment, I focused on people's thighs. They are big, easy to access, and all the thighs at this bike race were obviously working very hard. So I decided: At my checkpoint, I worked only on people's thighs. It was a good way to test the outcome of repeated, site-specific mini-Rolfing sessions. I knew that results had to be consistent to be valid. For example, I expected to find out that working on the fronts of thighs would be good for achy knees, for example, or bad for sore hamstrings, bad for painful ankles, and so on.

When I started, I had no idea what I'd find.

At one checkpoint, a cyclist complained of a sore hamstring, so I began Rolfing the front of his thigh. I remember him saying to me, "Oh, gosh! That got rid of the pain in my hamstring. How'd you do that?"

I wasn't quite sure, so I said, "It's a secret."

The next rider complained of calf pain, and again I did a Rolfing mini-session on his thigh. He, too, noticed an easing of the pain and asked, "How did you do that?"

"Can't tell you," I repeated. "It's a secret."

A few cyclists complained of back pain, and they commented that whatever I had done to their thighs had relieved their sore backs.

Based on the riders' reactions and pain relief, I began focusing all my attention on their thighs when they complained of back pain and leg aches. And for the most part, they all felt better.

A few weeks later, I got the same kinds of results at a health fair for senior citizens. Again, I tried the same approach. Mini-Rolfing the seniors' thighs relieved their complaints of lower back pain, sciatic pain, and leg pain.

Aha! Putting It Together

Over the next few years, I spent days in my office studying and analyzing anatomy charts, skeleton charts, and muscle maps of the human body. As I performed various bodywork techniques on clients, I would stare at the charts, trying to figure out why back pain and sciatic pain would respond to pressure and massage applied to the thigh. Why did two different types of pain respond to the same simple techniques? Why would a group of active, muscular cyclists get the same relief as a bunch of fairly sedentary senior citizens?

I worked with clients who were sincere and honest, the ones I knew who would answer my questions truthfully and honestly. I would do a technique and then ask, "What happened?" I avoided leading questions like "Did that help?" or "Is that better?" because I wanted to know specifically—nonjudgmentally, relevant or not—what was happening in their bodies. I was gathering information without pouring it into a mold. But like the cyclists at the race, all the clients told me that working on their thighs made their backs feel better.

After dismissing several theories, I settled on the concept of *position*. I realized that whether the body is actively working or passively sitting, the thighs are being shortened. It was this muscle-shortening, either by overworking the thighs or sitting for long periods, that affected the back.

Finally, the lightbulb went off. It was as if a voice inside me said, "I've got it!" What I got were the reasons the Rossiter stretches relieve back pain without ever touching the back.

Big Muscle/Little Muscle Phenomenon

One of the important concepts underlying the Rossiter back stretches is the interplay of big muscles and little muscles. Remember looking at anatomy charts in biology class and wondering if your body's muscles really looked like that under your skin? They do.

But one thing you might not have noticed is how muscles are grouped. Look closely, and you'll notice that each big muscle is paired with a smaller muscle. The strong, broad quadriceps muscle on the front of the thigh, for example, is paired with the skinnier hamstring on the back of the thigh. The biceps on the front of the upper arm is paired with a larger triceps on the back of the arm.

The back is supported by muscles all throughout the upper and lower body, but it receives primary support from two sets of layered muscles—stomach muscles and muscles on the back itself. These muscles provide support to the back, day in and day out. They provide balance to the body, front to back. They help the back do all of the actions it's supposed to do— stand, sit, walk, bend, lift, crouch, lean. . . .

The back also receives extra support from muscles and connective tissue elsewhere in the body—the head, hands, arms, neck, thighs, hamstrings, knees, calves, ankles, feet. But of all the leg, muscles that directly support the back, the most important ones are the thigh muscles.

The back itself sits atop an inverted triangular bone called the *sacrum*. It's one of the broad, rounded bones of the pelvis. The *femurs*, or thigh bones, stretch up to the back from the legs, and the pelvis rests on them. The heads of the femurs sit in sockets in the pelvis, and they act as fulcrums for balancing the upper body. All of the muscles that support the back attach to various points around the hip and pelvis, and connective tissue holds everything together.

The back balances around this swiveling, pivoting, sturdy structure, and doing so is a big job. From the hips, back, and pelvis, your body's muscles allow you to bend forward, squat, turn, lean sideways, curl into a ball, arch backwards, and swivel.

Back to the big muscle–little muscle phenomenon. "Big" and "little" involve more than size, because the bigger muscles aren't always that much larger than the smaller muscles, but God obviously wanted one to dominate in case of emergencies.

The bigger muscles all have similar jobs. They're designed to make joints open or extend, to help parts of the body move out and away by reaching. When you extend your arm and elbow to pick up car keys from the kitchen counter, for example, the bigger triceps on the back of the arm is activated to reach outward.

The smaller muscles do the opposite. They contract the joints, pulling the body back in toward itself. Using the same example, when you pick up your keys from the kitchen table, the smaller biceps is activated to pull your arm back to your side and plop the keys in your pocket. All of this is done in balance. Both sets of muscle control the speed, weight, and amount of reach during the movement.

The big muscles and little muscles are supposed to work in harmony. The body is meant to stretch and relax to a point that feels comfortable, loose, and easy, no matter what you're doing—standing, bending, rolling into a ball, crouching.

Big-Muscle Bully: One of the Thighs

The body can be like a playground: put big guys and little guys together, and the big guys always win. The bullies always bully, because they can. They're stronger and bulkier.

In your body, your big muscles are the big guys. They always win. They're always stronger and they always out-muscle the little muscles. In the back specifically, the muscles on the front of the thigh are the muscles that control the hip and pelvis (see figure 11.1). Look at any athlete's legs, and the front thigh muscles are always bulkier and stronger than the muscles of the backs of the legs. That's how they're designed.

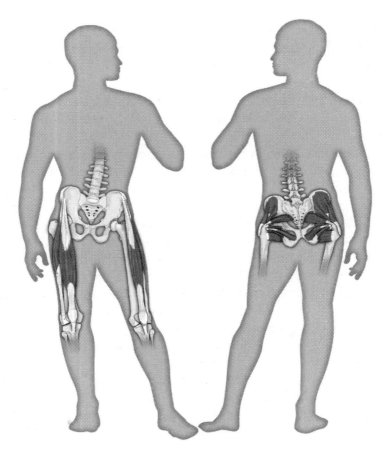

Figure 11.1   Big Muscle/Little Muscle

Look closely at figure 11.1. The muscles of this structure are exaggerated, but they reflect what happens when someone adopts the habit of constantly standing or leaning on one leg rather than the other. Over time, the muscles of the leg and hip doing the work become a little denser, thicker, bigger, and stronger. Again, sometimes the kind of work you do forces one side of your body to work harder or take more of the brunt of physical exertion, so muscles on one side get stronger and bulkier than the other side. Often, people say they lean on one leg because the other one hurts. In actuality, they've been standing that way for a long time and are now paying the price because they've changed the anatomy of their body's muscles and created an imbalance.

When you lift, the thighs are involved. When you turn, the thighs are involved. When you stand and lean on one leg out of habit, the thighs are involved. Each time they work, the thigh muscles contract and the muscle cells fire, shortening and tightening to give the muscle its strength and power. And when the muscles work, the connective tissue around them works, too.

Whenever the connective tissue of the thighs shorten, it affects the health of the back, usually with pain. Why? As you learned in part I, when connective tissue in any tense muscle shortens, it tends to stay shortened until a particular effort is made to stretch it back.

All the thigh muscles act as though they're attached to the hip at the anterior superior iliac spine, or ASIS on the front of the back's fulcrum. What develops is a teeter-totter, or lever, phenomenon (see figure 11.2). As the thigh's connective tissue and muscles tighten and shorten, they automatically rotate the pelvis forward and down in front (see arrows), causing the connective tissue and muscles on the back of the teeter-totter to be pulled upward. In other words, when the thighs tighten and shorten in front, they pull on and tighten your hamstrings on the back of the leg. This, in turn, tightens the back because of the forward rotation of the pelvis. In other words, that rotation causes the body to tilt forward. And to remain upright, you lean back, causing tension in the back.

When athletes complain of hamstring problems, it simply means the quadriceps muscles of their thighs have overdeveloped to the point that they're pulling the hamstrings way too tight to allow balance from front (thigh) to back (hamstring). Football players' thighs, even without pads, are huge. So are hockey players'. (Having been a hockey player of some repute, I can vouch for this. My high school yearbook notation: "Richard Rossiter wills his hockey skates to anyone who doesn't wish to play.")

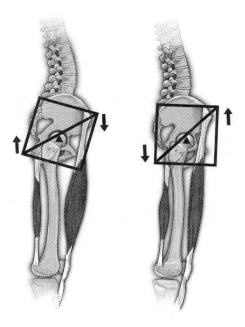

Figure 11.2   The Lever

To get a sense of the lever, try this. Take a rubber band and stretch it tightly around your thumb and forefinger. Make sure the tension is even on each side. That's how the back's muscle/connective tissue should be at all times—the same looseness on one side as on the other. In effect, it's balanced.

Now pull down or outward on one side of the rubber band. Stretch it out and tighten it. That's the equivalent of your strong thigh becoming tighter or tenser, exerting force on the rest of the back. See what happens? The tightened side becomes tenser, and your finger and thumb want to rotate toward the tense side. Not only do your fingers want to roll toward the tight side, the other side gets stretched. That's the equivalent of the muscles on the back of your leg and in your lower back tightening and pulling in response to your overpowering, tightening thigh.

Two Types of Back Pain

"Oh, the left side of my lower back is killing me!" "Oh, I have a pain shooting down the back of my right leg!" "Oh, I have a pain in my left butt cheek!"

How many times have you said—or heard—those phrases used to describe back pain?

That pain, as we've just learned, is the result of overworked or tense muscles and a shortening/tightening of the connective tissue that envelops the muscles of the thigh. In essence, the thigh's connective tissue is pulling the rest of the body out of its normal position, twisting, straining and pulling the muscles of the back and the hamstrings.

The pulling and tightening in the thigh causes the sensation of pain to appear in the back or the body or down the legs, when in actuality, the connective tissue imbalance starts in the thigh.

This imbalance isn't normal, but it's common. Most people at one time or another do this to themselves. How?

Most back problems are the result of muscle strains, bad habits, and lack of exercise. Bad back habits include the following:

- ▶ Poor posture

- ▶ Lifting/pushing too much at one time

- ▶ Lifting improperly or too intensely

- ▶ Leaning to one side more than the other

- ▶ Standing on one leg more than the other (Everyone does this. You do too, even if you're not aware of it. Next time you're standing in line, notice which leg you lean on most. And try to quit doing it. Share the load equally between both legs.)

▶ Using one side of your body more than the other, either by habit or by necessity (Maybe your work station forces you to turn, twist, or pivot only to the right, or only to the left. Maybe an injury causes you to rely on one side more than the other. Maybe you're compensating for pain by overworking one side of your body to give the other side a rest.)

▶ Tummy-butt-shoulders. Are you tight or relaxed?

Any of these habits can throw the back out of balance, and as you know when it becomes unbalanced, its basic components—nerves, muscles, and connective tissue—can't work properly, and they tighten, shorten, and produce pain.

How can you determine which type of back pain you have?

Type One

Type One is generally quick, acute back pain, usually from an injury to the back. It happens instantaneously. You bend over to pick up something, and you feel a tremendous shot or zing in your back. You slip and fall and hurt your back. You trip down the steps and whack your back. Sometimes, it happens so quickly that you can't breathe or you can't stand up. It's immediate and it hurts.

When you injure your back by lifting or bumping it on one side or the other, the action usually affects only that side. The pain exists where the injury occurred, and it can be felt in the immediate area of the back or it can shoot down the leg. When you use the Rossiter stretches for Type One pain, you stretch the thigh that's on the same side of the body as the pain. About 10 to 15 percent of back pain, in the Rossiter System experience, is Type One. As you'll learn in the next chapter, though, the Rossiter stretches assume that back pain is Type Two, because it's more common than Type One.

Type Two

Type Two pain develops over time. It's a dull ache. It's a pulling, tightness, or huge strain. It feels as if it'll be there forever, as if something has a nagging, painful grip on your back and will never let go. Then it does go away, and you can't figure out how or why. But it returns, like an annoying relative looking for a place to stay.

The reason that back pain is often more noticeable on one side of the body than the other, or why it feels like a slow thumping or throbbing sensation, is because of the *cranial-sacral pump*, a circulation system at work inside your body that's independent of the heart and lungs.

The Cranial-Sacral Pump

The cranial-sacral pump brings necessary fluid and nutrients to the spine and brain. You don't have to believe in it or remember it, because the cranial-sacral pump isn't generally known to laypeople or those in traditional medicine. It's discussed mostly in the field of alternative or complementary health. Chiropractors and body movement specialists refer to it a lot. The pumping happens, every day without fail, the same way your heart beats or your eyes blink, without conscious awareness.

In the Rossiter System experience, 85 percent of back pain is the result of an imbalance in the cranial-sacral pump and the resulting compensations people make to deal with their back pain. The cranial-sacral pump affects both types of back pain, but it's particularly a factor with Type Two pain. If you choose to treat your back pain with surgery or shots (injections) into the back, no matter what the diagnosis, pardon the frankness, but you're screwed. All backs degenerate over time. These stretches represent the least invasive techniques with the best results for back pain. So read on with the idea that these stretches will be able to help you. If you've already had back surgery, you can stop reading here—and do not do these stretches.

How the Cranial-Sacral Pump Works. Spinal fluid, or cerebrospinal fluid, is a nutrient-rich fluid that moves around the brain and through the spinal column, delivering food and oxygen to the delicate spine and nerves and taking away waste. The spinal fluid isn't static; it's constantly and regularly moving, up and down the spinal column, doing its delivery work and keeping the spinal cord healthy, nourished, and free of waste.

The pumping action is provided by your body's movement, a combination of the cranium contracting and expanding and the sacrum gently rocking, top to bottom. First, the fluid is whooshed from the cranium downward to the base of the spine. Then the sacrum (the triangular bone at the base of the spine) returns the flow by pumping the fluid up the spine. Without missing a beat, this pumping occurs about twelve times a minute and has a rhythm, or pulse, that can be felt by the naked hand. Two common activities—breathing and walking—enhance this action.

On either side of and attached to the sacrum are six very important muscles. As a group, they're called the *deep rotators*. These muscles attach to the upper end of the leg bone, or femur, at a place called the *greater trochanter*.

Remember the big muscle–little muscle phenomenon?

These deep rotators can become bigger or smaller than each other when you use your body in unbalanced ways. Think about the bad habit of leaning. Or working one side of your body harder than the other. Or twisting the same way every time. These movements, or habits, create the big muscle–little-muscle phenomenon from side to side in these deep butt muscles. It's not noticeable—you can't see that one butt cheek is slightly bigger than the other, but it's there.

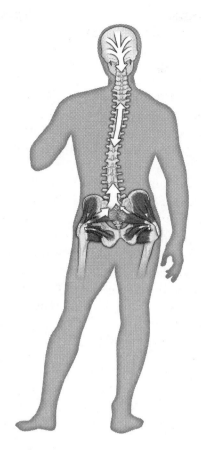

Figure 11.3 The Cranial-Sacral Pump

When muscles on one side of your body get stronger, they basically say to the weaker side, "You do all the work. You work the pump. You make this cranial-sacral thing work." So those opposite-side, weaker muscles become overworked, stressed, and tight—and that's why the sciatic nerve throbs. The deep rotator muscles that surround the sciatic nerve are being bullied by the stronger side. (In fact, when people report a throbbing pain down the back of their leg, it usually throbs at—guess what?—about twelve "pulses" a minute. It's the same rate at which the cranial-sacral pump pumps.)

This happens because when you compare both thighs, there's also a bigger and smaller thigh. Most bodies are like this. Many people have one foot larger than the other, and women frequently notice that their breasts are not exactly the same size.

My left leg, for example, is noticeably larger than my right leg, and it all goes back to a skiing accident years ago. I loved ballet skiing because it was graceful. Klutz that I was, I could "perform" on the slopes and not be noticed under goggles and layers of ski garb. With about two weeks of experience under my belt, I tried a spin on both skis on the slopes at Red Lodge, Montana. I was alone. I turned into the spin, and my skis split apart. Each leg followed its own ski. I heard a loud snap, fell in a puff of snow, felt the pain and yelled a very loud (expletive deleted). I rolled over into the view of an 80-year-old grandmother on skis who asked, "Are you hurt?"

I was definitely hurt, and my right knee and right leg were never the same. I avoided surgery and continued skiing, with one notable exception. I did all subsequent tricks on my left (and uninjured) leg. Even though I quit skiing fifteen years ago, my left leg is still bulkier than my right leg.

It's not necessary for one thigh or leg to be noticeably thicker or bulkier than the other. All that's necessary for Type Two back pain is to have more tension in one leg, or to use one leg more than the other.

For example, if your right thigh is more tense than your left thigh, it's going to pull harder and farther down in front as it tightens.

For Type Two pain, the Rossiter stretches focus on the thigh—the stronger thigh—that's opposite the side of the back or leg that hurts the worst. The stretches restore the body's structural balance by loosening the more powerful thigh's stronghold on the back.

Compensating

Type Two back pain is also often the result of compensating. Most people deal with pain by compensating. If one side of the back hurts, they'll lean to the other side or shift their weight to the other leg. If it hurts to stand, they'll sit. They'll lift or carry things differently, trying to get away from the achiness on the side that hurts most. When they compensate, they create Type Two back pain.

The more you perform tasks or work in an unbalanced way, and the older you get, the more pain you'll put into your body and back if you don't keep it balanced. The key is to rebalance your back whenever possible. The Rossiter back stretches will help your back find balance again.

A Long-Term Solution

The Rossiter System techniques are based on simple stretching concepts that restore balance to the back. By stretching connective tissue and releasing tension in thigh muscles that control the back, the Rossiter stretches give the back its necessary space—the freedom to move—without touching it. These stretches are like removing a one-sided body suit that's two sizes too small. Once you take off the cramped body suit, everything inside is freed and loose again, able to fill up the new space it has. When you stretch and relieve the muscle tension and connective tissue tightness that's causing back pain, you free up the back for flexibility and looseness again—and you take away the pain.

Even if back pain returns, the muscles and connective tissue that support the back continually can be stretched and elongated using the Rossiter System to restore mobility and relieve pain. Back pain, in essence, does not have to be a lifetime companion. Some people with back pain are told, "You'll just have to live with it," and that's simply not true. The Rossiter stretches help people take care of back pain simply, effectively, naturally, and on a continuing basis.

With all of these forces ganging up on the back—the overpowering thigh, the side-to-side imbalance across the hip from bad habits or work stress, TBS—you begin to understand how the back can become unbalanced and painful.

People who take this Type Two back pain to doctors are usually told the following: "Go home and rest it. Stay off your feet for a few days." Often, that simply makes the pain worse because it does nothing to address the imbalance that already exists. Staying off your feet makes the weak side even weaker.

What the back needs in this situation is an owner willing to stand up, relax his TBS, and walk. The back needs to be straightened and moved equally so the spinal-cord fluid can flow freely to both sides of the back, both buttocks, both legs. Pain shoots down one leg because it's on the side that's been beaten up and stressed. It needs to be exercised and moved so that both sides share the load.

It's like milking a cow. If all you do is squeeze one udder, that udder's going to get sore, and the cow's not going to be very happy, either. You get a lot more productive work—and a lot more contented cow—if you spread the work equally among all the udders.

Before you begin the stretches, read the next chapter, with its important precautions and tips for doing the back stretches properly.

Be Nice to Your Back: Quick Tips

What can you do right now to relieve back pain?

The best way to get your back into some sort of equilibrium is to walk. That's right—walk. Walking naturally balances the body's muscles and conditions the cranial-sacral pump. As you walk, relax your tummy-butt-shoulders (TBS). Here are some suggestions for incorporating walking into your daily regimen:

> ▶ Walk every day. Walk around the block a few times. Walk on your lunch hour. Walk to the market or bookstore. Walk just for the heck of it.

➤ Don't limp, or you'll make the pain worse.

➤ Swing both arms equally.

➤ Walk at least twenty or thirty minutes a day, if you can.

➤ Walk in shorts whenever possible to give your legs more freedom.

The following suggestions will also help you be nice to your back:

➤ Wear clothes that fit loosely and comfortably. Buy comfy, roomy jeans. Buy dresses and skirts that allow your body to move freely and without constriction.

➤ Wear low-heeled or flat-heeled shoes. Shoes with more than an inch heel throw your body off balance, setting in motion a tensing/tightening that causes back pain. Wear flats and sneakers, even if it means bucking fashion trends.

➤ Pay conscious attention to your body. When you feel it tighten, relax it. There are times to get wired, and times to unwind. Let the body use those unwinding periods to rejuvenate naturally.

➤ Relax your butt. Relax your stomach. Relax your shoulders. Take a deep breath and relax again. Doesn't that feel better?

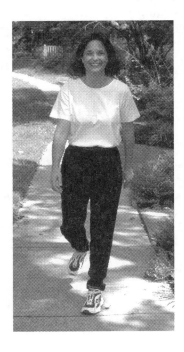

Figure 11.4   Walking

Chapter 12

Before You Start: Important Tips for Doing the Back Stretches

The back is an intricate, fragile but tough part of the body. Please abide by these guidelines to make the back stretches as safe as possible:

For the PIC

- ▶ Always do these stretches lying on your back, not on your stomach.

- ▶ Make sure to keep your hands on your stomach (a coffin position). That way the coach can watch your hands for signs of struggling, wincing, or pain.

- ▶ Do each stretch three times.

- ▶ If your back muscles begin cramping during any of these stretches, stop immediately. Wait a few minutes; if you want, start the stretches again where you left off.

For the Coach

- ▶ Never stretch someone who's had back surgery.

- ▶ Never stretch someone who's had cortisone shots or other kinds of pain-killing shots for the back injected directly into the back.

- ▶ Never apply weight to a person if large varicose veins are visible on the front of the thigh. If the PIC is wearing pants or slacks, ask about varicose veins.

- ▶ Do each stretch three times.

- ▶ Do not stretch someone who's had a broken bone in the affected area within the last six months.

- ▶ Do not stretch someone who's undergone a chiropractic treatment the same day.

- ▶ Do not stretch someone who cannot lie down on the floor. This seems obvious, but it may take some people ten minutes to get to the floor, and once there, they can't flatten their knees. That's a hint to not stretch.

Finding the PIC's Pain: The Rule of Three

As a coach, this may be the hardest obstacle you'll encounter with the back stretches, but your first job is to locate where the PIC's pain is. These stretches are done on the thigh that's *opposite the side of the back pain*, so in order to do them correctly, you first have to decide where the pain is. Then you know which thigh to stretch.

Always ask the PIC to locate the back pain three times. Why? I've had people tell me their back pain was in the middle of the back, show it to me with their left hand, and point to the right side of the back.

That's why it's important to ask three times, each time in a different way. It's the only way to truly pinpoint exactly what hurts and where. Asking three times gets the PIC to commit to a side. It weeds out wishy-washy answers. Asking three times gives the coach important and specific information. In the Rossiter System back program, all back pain is considered Type Two pain until proven otherwise, so it's important to start out accurately.

Once you find the most painful side, stretch only the thigh on the other side of the body. You'll get much better results, because you'll be working on the side that needs it and the PIC won't be moaning and sweating throughout the stretches.

If your PIC honest-to-God can't pinpoint the source of pain, don't do any stretches. The person probably is under the influence of drugs or is taking too many pain-killers to feel anything, and the stretches won't work. Even if the stretches were effective, you wouldn't know it because if the PIC can't tell any difference, you'll have a hard time convincing the PIC otherwise, even if you can see a change in how the person moves or stands. The Rossiter System stretches require active participation, conscious awareness, and persistence by the PIC, and good monitoring by the Coach.

How to Ask

All you have to do is ask, "Where does it hurt?" Most people will give you a clear indication of where their back hurts. It's a no-brainer. People with back pain will most likely point directly to the source of pain and tell you their story. Listen without judgment. If the PIC points to the upper part of the back or shoulders, do the upper-body workout from chapter 10 .

If the PIC points to the lower part of the back, keep an eye on three things:

1. **Which hand does the PIC use to point?** People with back pain almost always point with the same hand as the side of the back that hurts.

2. **Which way does the PIC turn his or her body in order to show you the pain?** People almost always turn the shortest distance to their pain to show you. If they turn to the right, their right side hurts. If they turn to the left, their left side hurts.

3. **On which leg is the PIC standing or leaning?** People who lean will lean on the leg that's most comfortable, meaning the opposite side of their back hurts. Stretch the thigh on which they lean.

    Some people swear they don't use one leg more than the other, so if your PIC is standing there describing the pain, note which leg she's standing on the most—but do not point this out. Just stand there and listen to the story. Some people will try to stand up straight, but eventually they'll slink into their habits, let down their guard, and lean. Watch for it. And as soon as you notice the lean, turn away and ask again, "Now exactly where is that pain?"

    Your PIC may look at you as if you have short-term memory loss, but all you're doing is verifying by behavior and stance everything you've been told verbally about the pain's location. (You can also ask a little differently, such as "Does it travel around or stay there?" In essence, you're forcing the PIC to pin down with consistency the location of the pain.)

So, your biggest indicators will be the physical habits and movements the PIC makes in describing the pain, moving, walking, and getting down onto the floor. Once on the floor, a PIC will usually keep the knee bent on the painful side, too. If someone's lying with the left knee bent, for example, the left side probably hurts more, so stretch the right thigh.

If the PIC describes the pain as "all the way across the back," ask the PIC to choose the side that's worse. It's the PIC's choice to make, even if it's switched from yesterday.

Which Thigh to Stretch?

This is important to remember. The back is unbalanced because one side is stronger than the other, and the stronger side is making the hurting side work harder. So by stretching out and loosening the stronger side, you're releasing its grip on the hurting side, and eventually the pain will go away.

If the PIC's back hurts worse on the left side, stretch the right thigh. If the PIC's back hurts worse on the right side, stretch the left thigh. It's that simple.

If you decide to stretch both thighs, follow these guidelines:

1. Stretch the thigh that's opposite the painful side first with a full series of stretches.

2. If you then decide to stretch the other side, you need to do only one-third as many stretches. For example, if you do three Windshield Wipers on the thigh that's the key to the PIC's back pain, do only one Windshield Wiper on the other thigh.

(Why? If you stretch both sides equally, the back will again be unbalanced. Remember, pain on the hurting side needs to be relieved more than it does on the less painful side.)

3. This applies to both Type One and Type Two back pain.

Adjusting for Type One or Type Two Pain

Once you start working on the thigh opposite the pain, one of two things will happen: the PIC's back pain either will ease after the first technique—or worsen. If the PIC isn't sure, standing up, walking around the room (no sauntering, no baby steps, just active walking), and comparing how his or her back feels compared to before the stretching started will help. Watch as the PIC stands up, notice if movement is different, and ask again if it feels better or worse. If it feels better, continue with the stretches.

If the pain feels worse after the first techniques, switch to the other side and begin working the other thigh. If pain intensified, it means your PIC has Type One pain. If so, stretch the thigh on the same side of the body as the pain. And remember, this is rare and it's usually the result of a recent injury.

A Word about Herniated Discs

Most people at some point in their lives will have back pain. But when you've been told you might have a herniated or bulging disc, you begin to see days ahead of no sex, limited activity, and surgery. Just the thought of surgery or something wrong with your delicate discs is enough—pardon the pun—to send chills up your spine.

There's good news and bad when it comes to herniated, bulging, or damaged discs.

The bad is pure awful. The Rossiter System is not recommended for anyone who's had back surgery or cortisone injections into the back. Keep in mind that 15 to 20 percent of people who have back surgery end up with more pain than they had before surgery, and some studies say up to 99 percent of back surgery is inappropriate, unnecessary, or unsuccessful for low back pain. In the Rossiter System experience, most back pain is a result of stressed and tightened connective tissue, and most of it responds to the stretches that loosen and free the connective tissue.

The good news is that you might not need surgery, and the disc problems might not be as bad as doctors make them sound.

I've worked with many people who've been told they had irreparable disc problems that required surgery. Some people opted for surgery, some didn't. Those who opt for surgery often assume that someone else can fix all their problems.

In my Rolfing practice and with these stretches, however, I've seen people get out of pain, be amazed, and leave happy—with no need for surgery. They proved to themselves—by doing the hard work themselves—that they needed to stretch in order to get rid of their back pain. They also learned not to let an outsider, myself included, manage their back pain because they understood it was their body and their responsibility to get rid of their pain.

If you loosen the connective tissue that is pulling and compressing on the spine, you loosen the pressure on the discs—the same pressure that may be making them bulge or balloon out. Loosen the pressure by stretching, and they quit bulging and hurting. If you're serious about taking charge of your back pain, get serious about these stretches. If you truly want someone else to manage your back pain for you, I'd much rather you see a chiropractor any day than have surgery. If you want to prevent back pain, use a daily stretching program like yoga to stay supple and flexible.

You're now ready to start doing the back stretches.

Chapter 13

The Rossiter Stretches for the Back

Reminders for the Back Stretches

As with the other Rossiter stretches, these back techniques require team-work, communication, and attention to detail.

Keep these tips in mind as you stretch.

- ► Keep breathing throughout.

- ► Keep your eyes open.

- ► Do the stretches very slowly and very deliberately.

- ► Do the stretches as a series, not individually. Do Gas Pedal, Wind-shield Wiper, Knee Up and Down, and Knee Circles in order. They get progressively more difficult, so it helps to start with the easier stretches first.

- ► Pay attention to your body and the signals it sends you.

- ► With all the back stretches, do the stretches on the thigh that's oppo-site the side of the back that hurts worse. If the PIC's worse back pain is on the right side of the back, stretch the left thigh (and vice versa). Typically, you should do the stretches only on one side of the PIC's body.

- ► The assumption is that the PIC has Type Two back pain. If so, stretch-ing the thigh that's opposite the back pain will relieve the pain. How-ever, if doing the stretches makes the PIC's back pain worse, the PIC probably has Type One back pain. If that's the case, simply switch to the other thigh and do the stretches there.

- ► All of these stretches use a 10-count for timing, but if the PIC wants to stretch longer, allow it. The PIC sets the pace and duration, depending on the amount of pain relief he or she is feeling.

Stretch One: The Gas Pedal

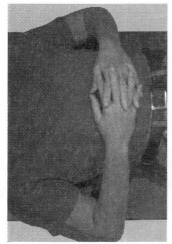

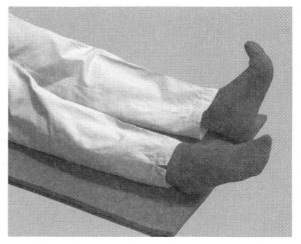

A   Hands on Stomach   B   Extended Foot

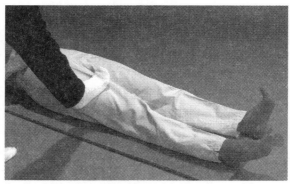

C   Pushing Out with the Heel

Figure 13.1   The Gas Pedal

What the PIC Does

1. Lie on your back on a mat on the floor. Relax. Put your hands on your stomach, palms down (as in figure 13.1A). Your hands can be inter-locking or not.

2. Your coach will place his foot high on your thigh and move it around slowly toward your knee, searching for knots or tender/sore spots on

the outer and upper parts of your thigh. Tell the coach when he's found the *most* tender spot.

3. After the coach has applied weight to that spot, Lock your other leg by pointing toes toward your head and holding the foot in that position. You should feel the Lock as a reach and stretch behind the knee.

4. Once you've Locked, your coach will begin a 10-count. Begin moving the foot of the leg being stretched forward (as in figure 13.1B) and backward very slowly, as if you're stepping and easing up on the gas pedal of a car. Stretch out the toes as far as they will point, then slowly bring them back in toward your body. As you draw your toes up toward your head, really push out with the heel (as in figure 13.1C). Hunt for areas of pain and stretch them slowly and deliberately. Step on the gas, push out with the heel. Make sure your other leg remains locked throughout.

5. When your coach reaches a count of 10, un-Lock and relax.

Hint: If you want to stretch longer, that's fine. Get in a really good stretch for whatever length of time feels comfortable. If this stretch makes you really whiny, stop at 10 seconds. If you feel it's doing a lot of good, keep it going until you feel satisfied with the stretch. Your foot should go forward and back at least three times during each repetition.

---

6. After the first stretch is over, the coach will apply his foot again to your thigh and begin looking again for the most tender spot. It may be the same spot, or it may be a different spot near the same place. Remember, the coach will ask you to tell him which spot hurts the most.

What the Coach Does

1. Ask your PIC to lie on her back on a mat on the floor. Hands should be placed on the stomach.

2. Place the arch of your foot on the outer part of the PIC's upper thigh and begin slowly pushing and adding weight downward, feeling for knots or tight spots on the thigh muscles. Continually ask your PIC, "Does it hurt worse here? Or here? Which spot is most tender?" You'll know where the spot is by paying attention to your PIC's words, reactions, winces, groans, ouches, or the way she tenses her hands. Some-

times when you find a really sore spot, you can move beyond it and continue searching. Sometimes you'll find even worse spots, sometimes not. Always go back to the one that makes the PIC wish for a trip to Tahiti.

Hint: This is what I call the "dentist's chair" phenomenon (figure 13.2). You'll know how much discomfort your PIC is feeling and how much effort she's putting into each stretch by watching how she grips her hands, grasps her fingers, or pinches her stomach.

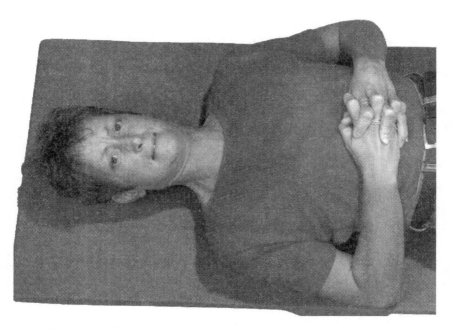

Figure 13.2   Dentist's Chair Phenomenon

Keep working toward the knee until you find the most tender spot. Stop at least 2 inches above the knee. There's no point in going farther. You should find the sore spot about two-thirds of the way up the leg, usually toward the outside of the thigh (see figure 13.1C). If you don't find a tender spot, start over. Apply more weight this time.

Hint: Stay away from the PIC's crotch, genitals, or anything that is sexual in nature—including inner thighs, nooks and crannies, zippers or bulges.

---

3. When you've found the most tender spot, add weight inward toward the bone (the femur) of the PIC's thigh. This motion will feel as if you are stepping downward or at an angle toward the center of the body. Add weight with the arch of your foot. If more weight is needed, use the area of your foot closest to the heel. Use the back of a chair for balance.

4. Ask the PIC to Lock by flexing the toes of both legs—toward the nose—and holding them there. Begin a 10-count now.

5. Now instruct your PIC to slowly, deliberately begin moving the toes and foot of the leg being stretched backward and forward. The toes should point down and away from the body, as if stepping on a gas pedal. When the toes return up, the heel should push out and away.

6. Make sure the PIC keeps breathing and keeps eyes open. Watch the PIC's eyes. Make sure she really stretches with the toes and pushes out with the heel. Look at her hands to see how hard she's working. And remember: It's all done very slowly.

7. When you reach a count of 10, remove your foot and ask your PIC to take a breath and relax.

Hint: It's okay to let the PIC stretch longer if she really feels the workout is doing a lot of good.

---

8. After the first stretch, use your foot again to search on the PIC's thigh for the most tender, painful spot. It may be the same spot or it may be a different spot. Just remember to continue searching for the worst spot, and keep asking questions until you find it. You'll do the stretch two more times. Each time, add weight at the most tender spot or knot on the thigh.

Bonus Back Tips for the Coach

Tip 1. Establish early that the most tender spot or knot is truly the most tender. If not, your stretching will not be effective. Usually, the spot you find the first time is indeed the worst one, but its location can change halfway through or near the end of a stretching session. Next time, follow it. It may divide in half or thirds. Always follow the most tender spot or knot—even if it's not the largest one.

Tip 2. The knot may try to roll out from under your feet when you add weight. Don't let it. If it starts to slide, change the angle of your foot to stop it and continue holding it until the PIC finishes stretching. This advice applies to all back techniques. Trap the sore spot with your arch.

Tip 3. Add weight steadily. Keep the foot steady while it holds weight in place. Don't let the PIC jerk, twitch, or pull away. If that happens, slowly remove your foot from the thigh and start over.

Stretch 2: Windshield Wiper

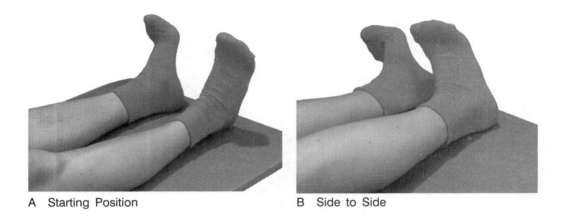

A   Starting Position   B   Side to Side

Figure 13.3   The Windshield Wiper

What the PIC Does

1. Lie on your back on a mat on the floor. Put your hands palm down on your stomach. Place your feet far enough apart that they are not touching and will not bump into each other. Relax.

2. Your coach will place the arch of her foot on the top of your thigh and begin searching for sore, tender spots or knots. Let the coach know when she's found the most tender spot.

3. After the coach has applied weight to that tender spot, Lock both legs by flexing your toes toward your nose and pushing your heels away from your butt (as in figure 13.3A). Your hamstring should be taut, but not too tight. Hold this Lock throughout the stretch. Keep checking to make sure your back is relaxed throughout the stretch. The coach will begin a 10-count.

4. Slowly and simultaneously move both feet back and forth, side to side (as in figure 13.3B), like a windshield wiper. Use the heel as a base for the wiper motion. (Moving both feet keeps them from clunking into each other.) Stretch into the pain. Do the side-to-side movements slowly, deliberately. Make sure the heels are pushing out and toes are pointed toward the nose. You can have just one leg move at a time or both (as in figure 13.4), but make sure the entire leg—not just the foot—takes part in the rotation around the heel. When the foot rotates in, the heel and the thigh should rotate in, too. In fact, the movement of the thigh (especially inward toward the body) is what makes this stretch so effective, so work the entire leg.

5. When the coach reaches a count of 10 (or longer, if you feel more time is needed for a really good stretch), un-Lock the legs and relax. Take a deep breath. Check and make sure your back is relaxed.

Get ready to do steps 1–5 two more times.

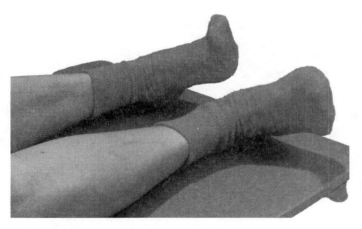

Figure 13.4   Two-Legged Windshield Wiper

What the Coach Does

1. Ask the PIC to lie on his back on a mat on the floor. Hands should be placed on the stomach. Make sure the feet are far enough apart that they will not bump into each other during the side-to-side movement of this stretch. The feet need at least a few inches between them.

2. Place the arch of your foot on the outer part of the PIC's upper thigh and begin feeling, pressing, and searching for tender or sore spots. Get the PIC's feedback on which spot hurts most. Ask your PIC to tell

you when you've found the spot that hurts the most or is most tender. Look for signs of tenderness—wincing, groaning, ouching, gripping hands. That spot is where you will add weight.

Hint: The PIC's hands are a good indicator of pain. They have a life of their own, able to impart information without the PIC even noticing. The fingers gnarl into a ball or make a fist that say, "You are seconds away from dying, Coach." That's the spot.

---

3. Add weight to that tender spot with the arch of your foot. If you need to add more weight, use the area of the foot closer to your heel.

Hint: It's a good idea to use the arch of your foot to start the feeling process because you can immediately start to apply weight to the tender area once found. This cuts out an unnecessary step and you become better at doing the techniques faster. The arch of your foot is very sensitive but untrained. Train it.

---

4. Tell your PIC to Lock with both feet by pulling the toes toward the nose and pushing away from the butt with the heels. Make sure the PIC keeps his back relaxed.

5. Begin a 10-count now and ask the PIC to begin moving both feet back and forth, side to side, in a windshield-wiper motion. Movement should be slow and deliberate. Make sure the heel is used as the base for the wiper motion, and make sure the whole window is washed. Tell the PIC to reach into the pain, and make sure the PIC rotates the entire leg, including the heel, foot, and thigh. The inward movement of the thigh is what makes this stretch so effective, so make sure the PIC is using the entire leg.

Hint: The PIC might not work as hard if the movement of the stretch is away from you. But moving that very area produces the best results with this technique, so really encourage effort in the stretch away from your body. Most back pain will be found in a sore knot or spot in the upper quadrant of the upper thigh, almost to the side of the leg. Find it.

---

6. Call the stretch finished when you've counted to 10 or when the PIC feels a really good stretch has been achieved. Ask your PIC to relax, un-Lock, and take a breath.

Hint: Sometimes you'll notice that one side of the wiper motion was not done as thoroughly as the other side. Guess what? The weaker side is the one that needs to be stretched the most. On the second stretch, make sure you encourage the PIC to work hard on the side that slacked off the first time. Don't let your PIC cheat. And get ready to watch some quivering!

To complete the Windshield Wiper set, do the stretch two more times. Each time move the foot to the most tender spot and add weight there. The exact spot may change during any of the back techniques, so continue hunting for the worst spot.

Stretch 3: Knee Up and Down

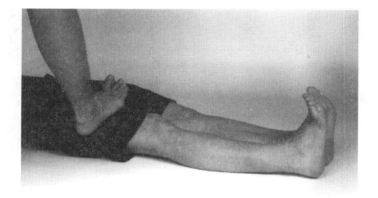

A   Start

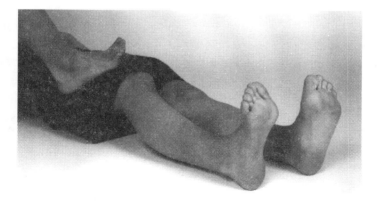

B   Up

Figure 13.5   Knee Up and Down

What the PIC Does

1. Lie on your back on a mat on the floor. Place your hands palms down on your stomach. Leave a little bit of space between your feet. Relax.

2. Your coach will place the arch of his foot on your thigh and begin searching for sore, tender spots or knots. Let the coach know when he's found the most sensitive and painful spot (keep your eyes open so the coach can tell by how much you're wincing!).

3. After the coach has applied weight to that spot (as in figure 13.5A), Lock both legs by pulling the toes toward your body and pushing out with your heel away from the butt. Hold the Lock throughout the stretch.

4. Using your entire stretching leg—not just your foot—turn the leg inward to about a 45-degree angle and hold it there. While dragging your heel and keeping your foot Locked, slowly pull and lift up your knee about 3 inches off the ground so that your leg looks like a very low pup tent (as in figure 13.5B). The important part of this stretch is what you'll feel underneath the knee and from the heel all the way up the back side of the leg. You especially will feel the stretch when you lower the leg to a flat and re-Locked position on the floor. Keep your heel pushed out. Move your foot and your knee at the same time and same speed. Reach with your foot and leg into the spot that hurts the most. Repeat the up-and-down movement of the knee off the floor several times (no higher than 3 inches) and return it to a flat, Locked position.

Hint: Keep the heel on the floor and let the heel slide along the floor while the knee is moving. Think of a Japanese fan; the bottom hinge is the starting point for each lift of the knee. Start by aiming the knee inward; then move up into the area where your knee was pointing. The second time, turn the leg and knee a little less inward and then move up into the area where the knee was pointing. Did it hurt more or less? If it hurt less, you're finished stretching in that area. Keep moving to a different rib of the fan. Each rib is another place to hunt for pain.

How can you tell if the Lock is still in place? Your heel will continue to stick out and away from the body. The back of the knee should feel stretched hard when the leg returns to the floor. Remember, do all movements slowly.

Warning! Do not use your back too extensively to make this stretch work or you will develop cramps in the muscles of your back. Stop immediately if the back starts to cramp! Relax, and then start over. If you develop cramps, you're involving the back too much and must go back to using only the legs. Do not tense your back during these stretches.

5. When your coach counts to 10 or calls the stretch over, relax your heel and take a deep breath. The coach will remove his foot from your thigh and begin searching for the next most tender spot. Again, it may be the same spot or a variation. The coach always searches for the most tender spot—the one that momentarily will make you miserable.

6. Get ready for two more repetitions. Relax and un-Lock between stretches.

What the Coach Does

1. Ask the PIC to lie on her back on a mat on the floor. Hands should be palms up on the stomach. Make sure there's a little bit of space between the feet.

2. Place the arch of your foot on the outer part of the PIC's thigh and begin feeling, pressing, and searching for tender or sore spots. Ask your PIC to tell you when you've found the spot that's most tender or painful. Look for signs of tenderness—wincing, groaning, ouching, gripping, or grasping the hands on the stomach. That is the spot where you'll add weight.

Hint: Wincing is good. Spastic jerking isn't good. If the pain is so intense that the PIC starts moving or wiggling out of position, stop, rest, and start again. If the PIC arches the back, start over. These stretches don't need to destroy egos. Some people can't tolerate as much weight, especially when they're learning these stretches and especially on a tender, sore knot. In many people, these knots really hurt.

3. Add weight to that tender spot with the arch of your foot. If you need to add more weight, use the area of your foot closest to the heel. Steady yourself with a chair because your PIC's movement may throw you off balance.

4. Tell your PIC to Lock by pointing the toes of both legs toward his body and pushing her heels out away from the butt. Make sure the Lock stays in place during the stretch.

5. Now tell the PIC to slowly turn the leg being stretched inward toward the body. Make sure the PIC turns the entire leg, not just the foot.

Hint: Be on the prowl for cheating. PIC's love to turn only the foot because it isn't as painful as turning the entire leg. This is an easy place for PICs to cheat if coaches aren't paying attention. So pay attention, and make sure the entire leg turns for this stretch.

---

6. When the foot is pointing inward at about a 45-degree angle, begin a 10-count and tell the PIC to slowly raise the knee up off the mat about 3 inches and then slowly send it back down to a position flat on the mat. The PIC's heel will slide along the floor to allow the knee to raise and lower. Remember, this is done very slowly. Tell the PIC to feel for the stretch that's occurring underneath the knee, from the heel all the way up the back side of the leg. If the stretch is done correctly, the knee and foot should be moving at the same time and same speed. Remind the PIC to keep breathing, eyes open.

7. Ask the PIC to repeat this up-and-down movement of the knee several times, reaching into the spot that hurts the most. Each time, the PIC's leg should raise in a slightly different spot to make sure the tender area is thoroughly covered and stretched.

8. After 10 seconds or several good up-and-down stretches, call the stretch over and ask the PIC to un-Lock and breathe.

Warning! Do not allow the PIC to use the back too extensively during this stretch. Doing so can cause cramps in the muscles of the back. Stop immediately if the PIC's back starts to cramp!

Do the stretch two more times. Each time, move the foot to the most tender spot and add weight there.

Stretch 4: Knee Circles

This stretch requires careful concentration by both PIC and coach, so stay focused.

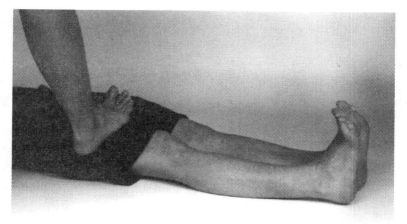

A   Start

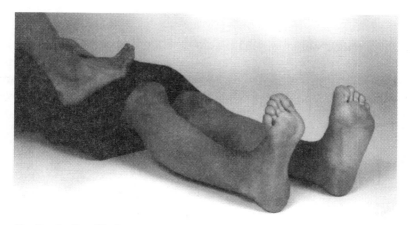

B   Begin the Circle

Figure 13.6 (A & B)   Knee Circles

What the PIC Does

1. Lie on your back on a mat on the floor. Place your hands palms down on your stomach, your legs slightly apart.

2. Your coach will place the arch of her foot on your thigh and begin searching for sore, tender spots or knots. Let the coach know when she's found the one that's most sensitive and painful.

3. After the coach has added weight to that spot, Lock both legs by flexing your toes toward your body and pushing out with the heels away

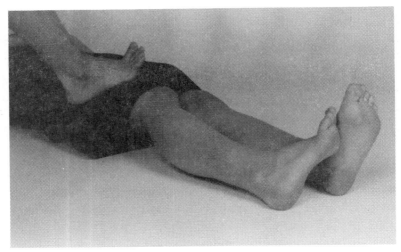

C   Inward

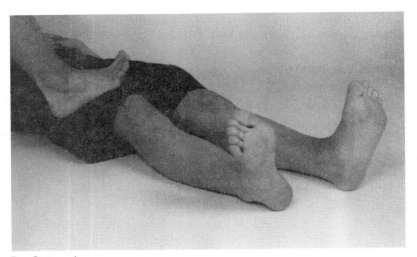

D   Outward

Figure 13.6 (C & D)   Knee Circles

from your butt (as in figure 13.6A). Hold that Lock throughout the stretch. Be prepared for this stretch, because it's more difficult than Knee Up and Down.

4. While the heels are Locked, slowly bring up your Working knee about 3 inches off the mat (as in figure 13.6B) and begin making a small circle, moving the knee inward (as in figure 13.6C), down, outward (as in figure 13.6D), and back up in a circular motion. Start making a circle with the knee from the bottom, with your toes pointing up.

On the downward and upward movements, you'll bend the knee as you feel the powerful stretch behind it. At the bottom of the circular stretch, your knee will again Lock, with the heel stretching to its maximum. You really need to feel this stretch on the back side of the knee. Reach into the spot that hurts the most in all areas. Do not cheat on this one. Don't avoid the pain and don't try to detour around it by making a smaller or incomplete circle.

5. When you've completed two full circles—clockwise and then counterclockwise—slowly take the knee back to the mat and let the leg lay flat. Un-Lock the heel and take a breath. Relax. This stretch supports all the previous work you've done in the legs and back, so don't slack off on this one. It's as if this technique makes the other back stretches complete.

What the Coach Does

1. Ask the PIC to lie on his back on a mat on the floor. Hands should be palms down on the stomach, legs slightly apart.

2. Place the arch of your foot on the PIC's thigh and begin feeling, pressing, and searching for tender or sore spots. The best spots for pain are on the outer quadrant of the upper thigh, near the groin. They are *not* in the groin, they are on the outside of the leg. A lot of these tender areas are almost lateral on the leg, so it may look as if you're moving your foot on the outside of the PIC's leg. Many times when you think you've found "the spot," you can move your foot a little more to the outside of the leg and find a more tender spot. For the PIC, that translates as "it hurts worse." Ask your PIC to tell you when you've found the spot that hurts the most or is most tender. Look for non-verbal signs of pain from your PIC. That tender spot is where you'll add weight.

3. Place the arch of your foot on that tender spot and add weight straight down. If you need to add more weight, use the area of the foot closest to the arch. Steady yourself with a chair, because your PIC's movements may throw you off balance a little.

Hint: If the PIC has thick legs, you may need to stand on something (a stool, a thick book) to raise your height a little so you can provide the amount of weight required.

4. Tell your PIC to Lock by pointing the toes of both legs toward the body and pushing out with the heels away from the butt. Make sure the Lock stays in place during the stretch. Keep a watchful eye on Locking, breathing, and making a full circle with the knee.

5. Now ask your PIC to slowly raise the knee no more than 3 inches off the floor, making sure the heel stays Locked. Once it reaches the up position (as in figure 13.6B), the knee should begin making a small 3-inch circle by rotating inward toward the body, then down and outward toward the up position for a complete circle. Repeat then rotate and make two circles in the opposite direction.

   During the rotation, the PIC will feel the stretch on the back side of the knee. At the bottom of the stretch, the PIC should be able to feel the knee re-Lock and should stretch the underside of the leg, all the way to the heel. Tell the PIC to reach into the spot that hurts the worst, both in the area where your foot is and in the part of the leg where he feels the stretch the most. If it seems as if the PIC is cheating, avoiding the most painful spot or making less-than-adequate circles, get some serious words of encouragement going.

6. After two clockwise and counterclockwise circles have been made with the knee, tell the PIC to return the leg to the mat, un-Lock the heel, and take a breath. Relax.

To complete a Knee Circles set, do the stretch two more times. Each time add weight at the most tender spot on the thigh.

Congratulations! You've now completed and experienced the power of the first level of stretches known as the Rossiter System!

For best results, go for a walk. It's the ideal way to help stretched-out connective tissue get some needed oxygen, nutrition, and blood supply.

Enjoy! Wiggle your tush! And notice how much better you feel!

Chapter 14

Why These Stretches Are Important: Ability, Capacity, and Adaptability

Most people who use the Rossiter System stretches like them—love them, in fact—because they produce instant results and get rid of soreness, aches, and pain.

But there are deeper reasons why the Rossiter System is important to individuals, companies, entire communities, states, and nations. The reasons all revolve around the issue of productivity.

The productive life of each person can be described in three words: ability, capacity, and adaptability. All three factors have powerful influences over each person's success of becoming a good worker.

Ability is an individual's aptitude or power to accomplish assigned tasks, physically or mentally.

Capacity is the amount of work an individual can do over a lifetime.

Adaptability is the amount of change an individual can endure throughout a lifetime of work, including mental and physical aspects of a job.

People are born with certain abilities. Most people have an ability for work, each in a different field. Some are good at mechanics or management, others at baking or piloting a plane. People who excel academically in life usually have more ability to work with their brains. They have higher capabilities to take on a variety of jobs that require thinking skills. With adequate education and experience, they become more adaptable and can choose from a larger pool of potential jobs or occupations. They are valuable to employers.

Adaptability is any worker's ace in the hole. It allows a worker to change as demands or requirements change, and adaptability is determined by several factors—education, experience, personal skills, and physical condition. A young tree trimmer, for example, can build on his skills and knowledge of tree-trimming. Then, as he ages and begins to doubt his ability to continue climbing trees with dangerous power tools, he can remain in the tree-trimming business by climbing down out of the trees to supervise others or to open his own tree business.

What does this have to do with the Rossiter System stretches?

On a very basic level, the Rossiter System is about helping one individual at a time out of pain. It's about you getting rid of the pain that's been keeping you from doing competent work, being happy, or feeling good inside your body.

But on a much broader level, these stretches address the serious issues of worker productivity, morale, pride, and capacity for work. On an even deeper level, they cut to the question of each company's, each community's, each nation's ability to compete and succeed in the world of business and work.

Here's one company's story:

"The Rossiter System works better than anything available anywhere today. It's a proactive approach that empowers people to get out of their pain," says Carl Rood, health resources manager and worker's compensation manager at Sauder Woodworking, an Archbold, Ohio, company that makes ready-to-assemble furniture.

Since adopting the Rossiter System in 1993 for its 2,600 employees, Sauder's worker's compensation costs have dropped precipitously. In pre-Rossiter 1991, the company paid $1 million in worker's compensation claims, a figure that has undergone a 51 percent reduction under the Rossiter System. The stretches have been particularly effective at reducing sprains, strains, shoulder injuries, and overexertion injuries.

"For years, the right thing to do has been to perform preventive maintenance on machinery and equipment and make sure they operate at peak performance," Mr. Rood says.

"But American industry has done just the opposite with our most important asset: our people. With employees, we work them until they break and then send them to a disinterested, third-party medical system and say, 'Here, fix them. We'll take them back when they're fixed.' If we continue with that approach, we'll never get rid of the injuries and disabilities that hamper our workers, impair morale, and slow productivity."

Based on the Rossiter System's early success, Sauder now has six full-time trainers available to provide stretching workouts to all company employees.

Says Rod, "In my seventeen years of dealing with worker's compensation issues and twenty-four years as a nurse, the Rossiter System stands out as the quickest, most effective way to bring under control overuse injury complaints, repetitive stress injuries, and everyday pain."

Capacity's Limits

A person's capacity to work grows, peaks, and declines with the condition of the human body. Laborers, assembly-line or factory workers, typists, office/computer workers, cashiers, keyboarders, fitness instructors are all people who rely on their bodies or parts of their bodies to perform work. They have a capacity to work that's entirely determined by how well and for how long their bodies can function free of pain, restraint, or limitation. Professional football players, for example, know they have a maximum of ten to fifteen years because their knees, shoulders, backs, throwing arms, or reaction times eventually will wear out, ache, weaken, or give out altogether.

Managers and decision-makers who understand the abilities and capacities of their workers will be the most successful managers. They understand that workers are not ideal workers if they are in pain, hurting, grumbling, or disenfranchised because no one understands the work they do or how much it grinds down their bodies. Workers in pain will not produce first-class products or reach optimum output. They will not be competitive. They will not care about the bigger picture. Most feel lucky just to get through the day.

In-the-know managers also understand that people who are pain-free—able to perform work capably and to their abilities—will work harder and better than those who ache or fill their bodies with painkillers, muscle relaxants, or other drugs to get by. It doesn't matter if you work inside your own home or inside a big company. If you are free of constant, chronic pain, you will work and feel better than someone who is plagued by it.

In essence, companies that grapple with repetitive-motion injuries, low morale, high absenteeism, soaring medical costs, and expensive worker's compensation claims actively need to find ways to make their employees healthier in order to maintain or increase their capacities and abilities to work. By doing so, the entire company becomes more adaptable to the winds of change and competition.

Managers who give their workers the resources to be free of pain are, in essence, giving them an extra hand to work. By contrast, companies that ignore their worker's injuries and pain are handicapping their employees. It's as if they're asking their own workers to do their jobs with one hand tied behind their backs yet compete with the office or factory next door, where employees can use two hands and have resources to stay pain-free while they work.

Why is this important?

Entire towns, cities, and communities rely on stable, productive work forces. States and nations compete with other states and nations for jobs. If one town's workers are hobbled by injuries that go unaddressed, employers look elsewhere, and when that happens, entire communities collapse. Tax bases dwindle. Schools become less successful. Community pride deflates. Native sons and daughters leave to work elsewhere.

The Rossiter System is one way for companies to keep their workers capable, adaptable, and able to fulfill their capacities for work.

Successful companies maintain their machinery and computers. Isn't it time someone turned attention to maintaining the flesh-and-blood, wage-earning human bodies that do the important work?

After all, without people, where would the machines be?

More Information About the Rossiter System

The stretches presented in this book represent the basic series of stretches developed by Richard H. Rossiter. The entire Rossiter System includes more than seventy stretches taught over eight levels, each level building on the skill, knowledge, and anatomy of the basic stretches.

If you or your company would like more information about the Rossiter System and how it might be able to help reduce worker's compensation claims and medical costs, improve worker morale, and get rid of or prevent workers' pains and injuries, please contact:

Rossiter & Associates, Inc.
1501 N. University Avenue
Suite 552
Little Rock, AK 72207
1-800-264-8100

Visit the Rossiter Web site at *http://www.rossiter.com* or call for information about stretching videos.

Join the Rossiter Revolution!

The Challenge of Scientific Research

By Ernst von Bezold

For whom will the Rossiter System work best and under what conditions? What else can be learned about and from the Rossiter System?

Program records show that about 10,000 people were doing Rossiter workouts regularly in 1998 in U.S. factories and offices. Firsthand investigation and interviews confirm that they use Rossiter techniques because they experience direct benefits.

Although the Rossiter System has not been studied extensively, two internal studies and one multi-year program performance review have been done by or for medium- to large-sized manufacturing companies that have implemented Rossiter programs on the job (von Bezold 1998). One of the studies is a clinical pilot followed by a case-matched retrospective comparison to physiotherapy (physical therapy). All have reported substantial net reductions, compared to case controls or historical data, in measures such as time off work and in all costs related to repetitive motion injuries (RMI).

This corroborates the clinical impression that the Rossiter workouts tend to provide participants with effective pain relief, support functional recovery, and help prevent further painful, potentially disabling injuries linked to repetitive motion.

The case of Sauder Woodworking provides an example of how worker compensation–related data can contribute to scientific assessments of the clinical and cost-effectiveness of a workplace program. At Sauder Woodworking in Archbold, Ohio (2,693 employees in 1997), workers' compensation costs for 1993 to 1997 showed a persistent net reduction of more than 50 percent, compared to the 1990–1992 baseline, within two years of implementing the Rossiter programs. The average dollar cost of RMI-related claims per employee hour worked, tracked by year of occurrence, was reduced from $.17/hour pre-Rossiter (1990-1992) to $.04/hour for the first three years of Rossiter programs (1993-1995). This 77 percent RMI claims cost reduction was accompanied by a similar drop in the number of RMI-related lost work days. Data for 1996 and 1997 confirm the improvement.

How likely is it that this reduction could be due to systematic error or to chance, i.e., arbitrary variations in the sample? There appears to be no evidence of a change causing bias in workers' compensation data. In addition to external factors such as inflation, two main factors affect the costs of RMI-related injury (immediate onset) and illness (gradual onset).

First, step-by-step ergonomic improvements should produce gradual reductions in RMI costs over time. Secondly, a growing, initially less-skilled workforce should show increased costs by the very nature of the workforce and the work.

Singly and together, these two main factors do not account for a sudden large drop in total workers' compensation costs over two years. In fact, the new Sauder baseline reached within two years of Rossiter implementation has remained substantially stable for the subsequent three years.

Data on individual employee costs is not available for calculating sample variance, so it is not possible to determine how much of the variation in average hourly injury costs is due to chance.

However, the number of employees is statistically large and growing: for 1990, N=1,510; the 1990–1997 mean average was 2,241. Sauder's workforce is also essentially permanent and full-time, providing a stable context for biostatistical analysis using individual workers' compensation data on file, such as days lost due to injury and illness.

Given the incremental ergonomic changes and attributes of the workforce, it appears that the size of the improvement in workers' compensation savings can be attributed credibly to the Rossiter System. It also is reasonable to anticipate that biostatistical analysis would support this conclusion. Research projects at this and similar sites have the potential to answer these and more specific practical questions about what works best for whom (USDL 1995).

Other Systems Corroborate Rossiter Results

Physical Methods

Published studies and treatment guidelines (State of Colorado 1998a, b) suggest that at least two other connective tissue–oriented systems are effective for RMI reduction.

A type of body work called Rolfing Structural Integration and a clinical soft tissue system called Active Release Techniques share a fundamental working principle with the Rossiter System. All three are designed to release adhesions between tissue surfaces by using weight or pressure to facilitate specific connective tissue stretches.

For the most part, medical and scientific literature takes connective tissue for granted when discussing cumulative trauma disorders or repetitive-motion injuries. When RMIs are not named specifically they are identified as "musculoskeletal disorders" (Bernard, Putz-Anderson, et al. 1997; Hasberg et al. 1995).

But a careful examination of the historical context of research and current scientific questions indicates ample, perhaps eventually compelling, grounds to broaden the paradigms for describing and treating repetitive motion–related injury, recovery, and prevention.

No matter how RMIs are defined, the cumulative weight of evidence for all three of these connective tissue–oriented modalities is strongly consistent with their specific claims of effectiveness for the relief and prevention of RMIs.

I have done a detailed comparison of the goals, effectiveness, costs, and benefits of these three connective tissue approaches with respect to RMIs. As part of that analysis, I have compared them with the current best practices in physical therapy (von Bezold 1998).

Overall, the connective tissue–focused modalities appear to be more effective clinically and economically than physiotherapy for rapid relief and long-term prevention of RMIs. The comparison included pain relief, restored functionality, development of resilience above baseline (indicating increased net wellness), the shift to user-based control of one's own recovery and prevention, length of training required, implementation cost, life cycle cost-effectiveness, and strategic value for a culture of wellness.

Learning-Based Strategies

The Rossiter programs' training and wellness orientation are mirrored less specifically but just as emphatically in the results of two remarkable programs for helping people recover from and prevent chronic pain and distress.

One is a managed recovery program for chronic pain sufferers called Educotherapy. Participants receive two weeks of classroom instruction in nervous system re-education, followed by ongoing home activity and telephone support. The program provides developmental, cognitive, behavioral tools that reduce or modify chronic pain and foster improvement in one or more of twelve other recovery categories, including immediate changes in the body's immune system.

The other is a drug harm reduction program sponsored by the ARTA Rehabilitation Foundation in the Netherlands. It provides recovering heroin addicts with specific learning opportunities to develop inner resources, especially individual life purpose, in a nutritionally and emotionally supportive environment.

Both systems demonstrate the practical effectiveness of the Rossiter strategy for teaching people to increase their health and wellness: build the workout participant's control of the process, reward personal initiative and effort with direct results, and help each other to progress and improve.

Research corroborates what experience shows (Fawzi et al. 1993): People who gain personal control over their own healing tend to take responsibility for improvement, take pride in their progress, see more immediate results, experience improved social independence, and are better able to deal with chronic overuse problems and pain.

The Rossiter System's synergy of physical effectiveness, self-determined quality of effort, and teamwork for progress in recovery and prevention offers a uniquely integrated, socially healthy model for building occupational well-ness.

Conclusion

Certainly learning more about the basis of the effectiveness of Rossiter programs will benefit the field of occupational health immediately. Medical and scientific literature already provides insights that can account for the paradigm-shifting innovations represented and integrated within the Rossiter System (Edwards 1993; Goodwin 1996).

Beyond that, diverse research indicates that an improved understanding of systemic functions of connective tissue in human biology has profound implications for basic health in relation to chronic diseases and aging. So does an understanding of experience-based developmental learning for wellness.

Connective tissue and wellness learning are both key elements of the Rossiter System. What much current research illustrates profoundly is that these two elements are also keys to understanding how we form our bodies. Do we form them well or not so well? Do they become arthritic, cancerous, or hobbled by heart disease, or do they remain fluid, free of cancer, and heart-healthy? Similarly, how do our bodies age? Quickly or slowly? Voluntarily or involuntary? How do we age, and how well?

Goethe suggested that loving something means that you come to know it. Perhaps this learning principle expresses the ultimate healing connection we may make with life through activities such as the Rossiter connective tissue workouts.

References

The references include Internet-accessible RSI and research funding resources. I gratefully acknowledge helpful discussions with epidemiologist Harry Shannon of McMaster University, statistician Chris Springer of the University of Waterloo, and analyst Jim Barnhardt of the U.S. Bureau of Labor Statistics.

Bernard, Bruce P., editor, and V. Putz-Anderson et al. 1997. Musculoskeletal disorders and workplace factors: A critical review of epidemiologic evidence for work-related musculoskeletal disorders of the neck, upper extremity, and low back [second printing]. U.S. Department of Health and Human Services Public Health Service Centers for Disease Control and Prevention National Institute for Occupational Safety and Health, July 1997; DHHS (NIOSH) Publication No. 97–141. NIOSH Publications

Dissemination, 4676 Columbia Parkway, Cincinnati, OH 45226-1998 USA. 1-800-356-4674. http://www.cdc.gov/niosh/homepage.html

Edwards, Lawrence. 1993. *The Vortex of Life: Nature's Patterns in Space and Time*. Floris: Edinburgh

Fawzi, F. I., et al. 1993. Malignant melanoma effects of an early structured psychiatric intervention, coping and affective state on recurrence and survival 6 years later. *Arch Gen Psychiatry* 50. Sept. 681–89.

Goodwin, Siana. 1996. *Rolfing for Work-Related Repetitive Motion Injuries*. Boulder, Colo.: Rolf Institute for Structural Integration.

Hagberg, Mats, et. al., authors, and I. Kuorinka, L. Forcier, scientific editors. 1995. *Work Related Musculoskeletal Disorders (WMSDs): A Reference Book for Prevention*. London: Taylor & Francis.

State of Colorado Department of Labor and Employment. 1998a. Workers' compensation rules of procedure 7 CCR 1101-3 upper extremity medical treatment guidelines v. cumulative trauma disorder (3/15/98 RMI V). Available through: Public Records Corporation, 171 17th Street, Ste. 1620, Denver, CO 80202. (303) 292-2575.

————. 1998b. Quick reference guide to be used in conjunction with upper extremity medical treatment guidelines cumulative trauma disorder. Revised March 15, 1998.

United States Department of Labor, Bureau of Labor Statistics. 1995. Workplace Injuries and Illnesses in 1995 [annual survey of occupational injuries and illnesses]. Internet address: http://stats.bls.gov/oshhome.htm.

von Bezold, Ernts. 1998. *The Rossiter System: Resources for Research*. Little Rock, Ark.: Rossiter and Associates, Inc.

References

American Academy of Orthopaedic Surgeons. 1999. "Lift It Safe" patient education brochure. AAOS, 6300 N. River Road, Rosemont, IL, 60018-4262, (847) 823-7186.

Eckel, Robert H., and Ronald M. Krauss. 1998. American Heart Association call to action: Obesity as a risk factor of coronary heart disease. *Circulation*. 2 June.

Fried, John J., and Sharon Petska. 1995. *The American Druggist's Complete Family Guide to Prescriptions, Pills & Drugs*. New York: Hearst Books.

Jerome, John. 1987. *Staying Supple: The Bountiful Pleasures of Stretching*. New York: Bantam.

Larson, David (ed.). 1996. *The Mayo Clinic Family Health Book*. New York: William Morrow Co. Inc.

Lazarou, Jason, et al. 1998. Incidence of adverse drug reactions in hospitalized patients. *Journal of the American Medical Association*. 279(15): 1200–1205.

Margolis, Simeon (ed.). 1995. *The Johns Hopkins Medical Handbook*. New York: Rebus Inc.

Mayo Clinic. 1994. Steroids. *Mayo Clinic Health Letter* 12(9). September. Rochester, Minn.

McTaggart, Lynne. 1998. *What Doctors Don't Tell You*. New York: Avon Books.

Medical Economics. 1998. *Physicians' Desk Reference*, 52nd edition. New Jersey: Medical Economics Co.

Oppenheim, Mike. 1994. *100 Drugs That Work: A Guide to the Best Prescription & Non-Prescription Drugs*. Los Angeles: Lowell House.

Potts, Laura. 1997. OSHA urges rule on repetitive stress injury: New study finds that injuries account for 62 percent of work-related illnesses. *The Detroit News*. 2 July. B-1.

Swoboda, Frank. 1997. Repetitive stress injuries are job reality, report says. *The Washington Post*. 2 July. D-11.

Tortora, Gerard J., and Nicholas P. Anagnostakos. 1984. *Principles of Anatomy and Physiology*, 4th edition. New York: Harper & Row.

More New Harbinger Titles

Some Other New Harbinger Self-Help Titles

Claiming Your Creative Self: True Stories from the Everyday Lives of Women, $15.95
Six Keys to Creating the Life You Desire, $19.95
Taking Control of TMJ, $13.95
What You Need to Know About Alzheimer's, $15.95
Winning Against Relapse: A Workbook of Action Plans for Recurring Health and Emotional Problems, $14.95
Facing 30: Women Talk About Constructing a Real Life and Other Scary Rites of Passage, $12.95
The Worry Control Workbook, $15.95
Wanting What You Have: A Self-Discovery Workbook, $18.95
When Perfect Isn't Good Enough: Strategies for Coping with Perfectionism, $13.95
The Endometriosis Survival Guide, $13.95
Earning Your Own Respect: A Handbook of Personal Responsibility, $12.95
High on Stress: A Woman's Guide to Optimizing the Stress in Her Life, $13.95
Infidelity: A Survival Guide, $13.95
Stop Walking on Eggshells, $14.95
Consumer's Guide to Psychiatric Drugs, $16.95
The Fibromyalgia Advocate: Getting the Support You Need to Cope with Fibromyalgia and Myofascial Pain, $18.95
Healing Fear: New Approaches to Overcoming Anxiety, $16.95
Working Anger: Preventing and Resolving Conflict on the Job, $12.95
Sex Smart: How Your Childhood Shaped Your Sexual Life and What to Do About It, $14.95
You Can Free Yourself From Alcohol & Drugs, $13.95
Amongst Ourselves: A Self-Help Guide to Living with Dissociative Identity Disorder, $14.95
Healthy Living with Diabetes, $13.95
Dr. Carl Robinson's Basic Baby Care, $10.95
Better Boundaries: Owning and Treasuring Your Life, $13.95
Goodbye Good Girl, $12.95
Being, Belonging, Doing, $10.95
Thoughts & Feelings, Second Edition, $18.95
Depression: How It Happens, How It's Healed, $14.95
Trust After Trauma, $15.95
The Chemotherapy & Radiation Survival Guide, Second Edition, $14.95
Surviving Childhood Cancer, $12.95
The Headache & Neck Pain Workbook, $14.95
Perimenopause, $16.95
The Self-Forgiveness Handbook, $12.95
A Woman's Guide to Overcoming Sexual Fear and Pain, $14.95
Don't Take It Personally, $12.95
Becoming a Wise Parent For Your Grown Child, $12.95
Clear Your Past, Change Your Future, $13.95
Preparing for Surgery, $17.95
The Power of Two, $15.95
It's Not OK Anymore, $13.95
The Daily Relaxer, $12.95
The Body Image Workbook, $17.95
Living with ADD, $17.95
When Anger Hurts Your Kids, $12.95
The Chronic Pain Control Workbook, Second Edition, $17.95
Fibromyalgia & Chronic Myofascial Pain Syndrome, $19.95
Kid Cooperation: How to Stop Yelling, Nagging & Pleading and Get Kids to Cooperate, $13.95
The Stop Smoking Workbook: Your Guide to Healthy Quitting, $17.95
Conquering Carpal Tunnel Syndrome and Other Repetitive Strain Injuries, $17.95
An End to Panic: Breakthrough Techniques for Overcoming Panic Disorder, Second Edition, $18.95
Letting Go of Anger: The 10 Most Common Anger Styles and What to Do About Them, $12.95
Messages: The Communication Skills Workbook, Second Edition, $15.95
Coping With Chronic Fatigue Syndrome: Nine Things You Can Do, $13.95
The Anxiety & Phobia Workbook, Second Edition, $18.95
The Relaxation & Stress Reduction Workbook, Fourth Edition, $17.95
Living Without Depression & Manic Depression: A Workbook for Maintaining Mood Stability, $18.95
Coping With Schizophrenia: A Guide For Families, $15.95
Visualization for Change, Second Edition, $15.95
Angry All the Time: An Emergency Guide to Anger Control, $12.95
Couple Skills: Making Your Relationship Work, $14.95
Self-Esteem, Second Edition, $13.95
I Can't Get Over It, A Handbook for Trauma Survivors, Second Edition, $16.95
Dying of Embarrassment: Help for Social Anxiety and Social Phobia, $13.95
The Depression Workbook: Living With Depression and Manic Depression, $17.95
Men & Grief: A Guide for Men Surviving the Death of a Loved One, $14.95
When Once Is Not Enough: Help for Obsessive Compulsives, $14.95
Beyond Grief: A Guide for Recovering from the Death of a Loved One, $14.95
Hypnosis for Change: A Manual of Proven Techniques, Third Edition, $15.95
When Anger Hurts, $13.95

Call **toll free, 1-800-748-6273,** to order. Have your Visa or Mastercard number ready. Or send a check for the titles you want to New Harbinger Publications, Inc., 5674 Shattuck Ave., Oakland, CA 94609. Include $3.80 for the first book and 75¢ for each additional book, to cover shipping and handling. (California residents please include appropriate sales tax.) Allow two to five weeks for delivery.

Prices subject to change without notice.